Hair Today, Gone Tomorrow

Hair Today, Gone Tomorrow
What I Lost and Gained Through Breast Cancer

Camy Crank

Copyright © 2022 Camilla Crank
All rights reserved.

Published by Calvary University Press
15800 Calvary Road
Kansas City, MO 64147
www.calvary.edu

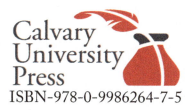

ISBN-978-0-9986264-7-5

Scripture quotations taken from the (NASB®) New American Standard Bible®, Copyright © 1960, 1971, 1977, 1995 by The Lockman Foundation. Used by permission. All rights reserved. www.lockman.org

Dedication

For you, my new friend, who have found yourself in a club you didn't choose to join, please, please know there is Hope.

Table of Contents

Chapter 1: The Unwanted Journey 1

Chapter 2: The Mom Becomes the Child 13

Chapter 3: God is Good 24

Chapter 4: Family and Such 33

Chapter 5: Time Well Spent 43

Chapter 6: Removal 51

Chapter 7: Thorny Ways Lead to a Joyful End 61

Chapter 8: Reconstruction 68

Chapter 9: Treasures Hidden in the Darkness 83

Chapter 10: Learning to Live Again 90

Chapter 11: God is Still Good 98

Chapter 12: Though I Walk Through the Valley of the Shadow of Death ... 115

Appendix A: Cancer Timeline 125

Appendix B: Memory Verses for Battling Cancer 132

Acknowledgments

I finished this book two years ago in November 2019—or so I thought! A few months prior while having lunch with my daughter-in-law, Krista, I mentioned I was almost done writing my book. Krista casually asked, "Are you planning to have someone proof it for you?"

"Yes, I replied—you." She and my son both have degrees in English, so I was hoping to include their expertise in my project.

Krista, thank you for graciously agreeing to my request. When we met later after your first read-through and you stated, "This is good and worthy of going to print, but I think it needs a complete overhaul," I was slightly overwhelmed at the fresh work ahead of me. Afterwards, though, when I looked over your detailed recommendations I knew you were right. I began writing again with vigor, appreciative that you would tell me your true opinion. With your advice my book became a more readable story.

After Krista and I went back and forth with the transcript a few times, I passed my book on to Thomas, my oldest child, Krista's husband, and college English professor. Thomas, with your tremendous creativity and extensive tutoring experience, you were able to draw out distinctive details of my story that I didn't even realize were missing. You are a grammar guru, using terms I can't define but definitely needed for the accuracy of my finished product. Thank you for applying your publishing knowledge to put my book into a print format. Thomas and Krista, my expert editors, from the bottom of my heart, I thank you.

Thomas helped me establish a publisher. Thank you, Calvary University Press for taking a chance on me.

I am forever grateful to my life partner and husband, Bob, not just for living my story with me, but making it clear that you are here for me 'til the end.

Thanks to my youngest child and nurse, Meridith; you wrote part of my story as you walked with me into my diagnosis.

Thank you, Bob and Meridith, for being my very first readers early on, correcting numerous errors and offering solid suggestions.

A huge thank you to my middle child and Naval Officer, Kevin. Kevin, your encouragement to write a book, assuring me that there were many readers of this genre got me serious about seeking to publish my work.

Thank you to the skilled doctors, sensitive nurses, friendly medical workers, and pleasant employees who have taken care of me at The University of Kansas Health System. You are concerned about my whole person, giving expert treatment, hearing my questions, and comforting me during procedures. I consider you my friends.

Many thanks to my extended family and friends who are a part of my story. You will see yourself in these pages. Thank you for continuing to be interested, asking about the progress of my book, and believing I could finish it.

I'm eternally grateful to God for His forgiveness of my sins so I can be His child and have a home in Heaven forever. Thank you, God, for giving me Your grace to walk this road and for never leaving me. God is writing my life's story, and He is the One who gave me the ability to tell it back to you. All glory be to God.

Preface

When I came face to face with the possibility that I had breast cancer, I came undone. I became scared of the dark and could only sleep with praise music playing through my iPod earbuds or curled up in my husband's arms. I became a recluse, not wanting to see or talk to anyone, not wanting to go anywhere—not even church, which previously had been my solace. I didn't want my phone near me; it startled me with its rings and tones. I cried a lot. Our daughter, Meridith, bore the role of my secretary, appointment maker, care giver, and encourager.

I repeated Isaiah 41:10 over and over for comfort, following each phrase with my own prayer:

> "Do not fear,
> *[I am afraid-God, please help me.]*
> for I am with you;
> *[Thank You that You are here.]*
> do not anxiously look about you,
> *[I am anxious and suspicious, Lord!]*
> for I am your God.
> *[Yes, You are my God.]*
> I will strengthen you, surely I will help you,
> *[I can't feel Your help right now, but I will trust in Your true Word.]*
> surely I will uphold you with My righteous right hand."
> *[Your hand is all powerful. I can rest knowing You do what is right.]*

Though the Bible was the greatest source of comfort to me, I also sought out books about people who had traveled this road before me. I scoured our library's portal, searched elsewhere online, and asked for recommendations from friends. After I read the few books I found about breast cancer survivors, I expanded my repertoire to any autobiography of survival. I needed inspiration. I needed to hear from someone I could relate to and glean hope from.

As I was recovering from breast cancer treatment, I decided to write the book I wish I could have read at the start of my cancer journey, a book filled with spiritual and emotional encouragement for fellow cancer patients. I wanted to include the raw gamut of my continually changing feelings, to take the reader into my journey from appointments and tests and procedures, and lastly to offer hope on how to cope with this life-altering diagnosis. My family rallied around my idea of writing a book, so I began collecting notes in the "Notes" app of my iPhone and iPad. I tapped out notes in the waiting room, on the couch before bed, during vacations, and in any free moment when I got an idea.

In September of 2019, now four years into writing my book, I was visiting my daughter in Minnesota. I had a few minutes to work, so I opened my iPad to put the finishing touches on the first two chapters when the unthinkable happened: they had disappeared! I had previously purchased iCloud storage, assuming my notes were backed up, so I quickly opened my iPhone, but they weren't there either. My daughter, who is more adept in computers than I am, assisted me for over an hour. We travailed to no avail. We called Apple support, continuing to move up the chain of command to more knowledgeable technicians. Finally, Apple submitted a claim to their research department.

Five days later I was back at home when I received the follow-up call from Apple. There was nothing they could do to bring back my two missing chapters. Apparently, there was a fluke in their system, and, despite having selected my notes to be stored in iCloud, they were saved in Yahoo, our email service provider. Contacting Yahoo yielded same news: no notes.

I was physically numb and couldn't do anything the rest of that day. I remember talking out loud to God about it, pacing back and forth, wandering through the whole house. I thought to myself, *All this hard work, and now it's down the drain!* I wondered if I shouldn't write this book after all. I examined my heart. Were my motives pure in wanting to publish a book? I recommitted the book to the Lord, reminding myself that if I did continue to write it, all the glory would go to Him. I went to bed that night deciding to give writing a break and pursue other interests for a while.

The next morning, I awoke to find a smattering of printed pages at my place on the breakfast table. I couldn't help but notice the headings "Chapter 1" and "Chapter 2"! *What in the world?!* On another page was scribbled in my husband's handwriting:

Your notes are in Yahoo Notes. All seem present. Please save them somewhere.

Praise the Lord!! God brought back your notes as only He can do.

Now, write your book, my Dear.

Love you,
Bob

The book was on!

It is my prayer that this book provides you with practical help through the cancer journey, encourages you through the wisdom and comfort of God's Word, and draws you closer to our Savior Jesus Christ, the Author and Finisher of our faith.

> *"Now to the King eternal, immortal, invisible, the only God, be honor and glory forever and ever. Amen."*
> *– 1 Timothy 1:17*

You may contact me at camycrank@gmail.com.

CHAPTER 1

The Unwanted Journey

I have always thought my hair was my best feature. I have had long hair as long as I can remember. "The reason I have so many boyfriends is because they like my long hair," I once told my parents. When I was older, my sisters said they wished they had thicker hair like mine. Often, mere strangers would stop me to tell me how pretty my hair was. My hair was my crown.

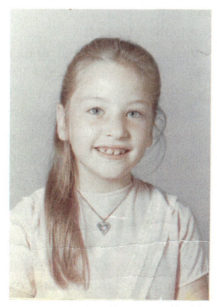

Me in 2nd grade.

Under the hair, I am a very predictable person, bordering on boring. Unlike a sister who tries something new every year—book of the month club, state hiking group, women's tournament fishing—there are no big adventures for me. I don't need to make New Year's resolutions, as I do the same thing every year—that is, until one quiet night in January 2015 when my husband, Bob, found the lump in my right breast. This began a journey that resulted in the loss of my hair and the scattering of my scheduled life. I barely recognized myself for a time, but this was also a journey of God's grace, and though I didn't want the journey, what I gained out-weighed what I lost.

Bob urged me to get the lump checked out, so I made an appointment as soon as my schedule would allow. I had faithfully gotten annual mammograms for years, never having a suspicious area yet. I was convinced this new-found lump was just another pre-menopausal symptom, as the last few years my periods were going back and forth from skipping to gushing as my body was trying to make the transition to menopause. My primary care physician (PCP) had ordered a cervical biopsy December 2013, which came back negative. I assumed this would have the same outcome.

When I saw my PCP about the lump, she scheduled a breast sonogram and diagnostic mammogram (even though I had just had my yearly mammogram in October, which was normal). A few days later I received a call from my PCP's medical assistant (MA), telling me the tests were negative and to repeat the mammogram in a year.

"A year from last October or a year from now?" I asked.

"A year from now," she replied. Nothing was said about doing a biopsy. It didn't even cross my mind to ask for one. Since then, I have discovered that many of my friends have had breast biopsies, as that is the surest way to know if the suspected area is cancerous or not.

Fast forward a few months—this "non-cancer" kept growing, so we decided we were not going to wait a year to get it checked again. My nipple was now becoming inverted and had developed a smelly discharge. I again made an appointment with my PCP.

She started with cheery small talk, but as soon as I opened my gown, she stopped mid-sentence, a look of horror on her face. I have never seen a doctor look this way before; they are usually so in control and emotionless. She grabbed a tape measure, exclaiming, "I thought I told you to get a sonogram and diagnostic mammogram?!" She was now talking to my breast as she measured the object of her focus, the menacing lump.

I don't know if she cared to know my answer, or if she even heard my response, "I did go for the referred diagnostic mammogram and sonogram.

After receiving the results, your MA called telling me everything was okay."

"Well, they were wrong! They were wrong!" She promptly ordered a repeat of the two tests.

When I emerged from the exam room, my PCP, who was whispering to the authorization clerk, suddenly quieted herself and left. The authorization clerk scheduled the two tests for the following day, apparently fitting me into an already full schedule. I felt ashamed, as if I had not followed the doctor's orders, when in reality, I came in several months sooner than was suggested.

I returned the next day, a Friday afternoon. I wanted to get this over with, fully expecting a repeat performance of a few months prior.

Boy was I wrong!

The mammographer made small talk as she started the scan, saying she remembered me from January. Her demeanor changed as she studied the screen. She scurried out the room without saying a word to me. When she returned, she avoided eye contact, told me to get dressed and wait in the main waiting room again until they were ready for the sonogram.

It was like being in a horror movie. It was like she and my doctor were on the same script. I had become a non-person, apparently with a medical problem, that they were uncomfortably trying to deal with. It sent shivers through me. I was physically shaking. All I had on was this light gown in an air-conditioned room—made extra cold for the machinery. All my muscles were tense. The physical discomfort mirrored my emotional feelings. No one at this facility ever said the word *cancer* to me. *Tell me what's going on,* I thought. It was like they had knowledge they either didn't know how to tell me or didn't want me to know.

After being called back for the sonogram and getting undressed again, we began going through the same sequence as five months ago.

"I've seen enough, I'm coming in!" a male voice shouted. A man barged into the room, and there I was lying on the table, breasts fully exposed, now with a stranger staring down at me. "You have an area that needs an immediate biopsy," he said as if I were the problem and had neglected my health and avoided getting medical attention.

"Excuse me," I said. "Who are you?"

"I'm a doctor," he said. Then, looking down, he realized he didn't have on his name tag.

"Uh, okay," I said. Then with a trembling voice I continued, "Do you want to do the biopsy now?"

He looked annoyed. "I can't do that now," he muttered. "I've already stayed overtime as it is. Any one of my *colleagues* are qualified to do this." It became obvious that I was "worked in" on this Friday afternoon and was messing up everyone's weekend plans.

I later wondered if possibly this doctor was trying to put the blame on me as he knew it was their fault they hadn't biopsied this place in my breast months ago. This was the hospital where I had had all my previous annual mammograms. They had my full medical records. I had followed all their protocols.

I received pity instead of compassion—techs with averted eyes afraid to connect emotionally with me, trite comments instead of genuine concern. No one even had the courage to tell me I might be dealing with cancer. I was treated like I was a germ. I couldn't get out of there fast enough!

I got dressed and left, wishing these awful events could be erased from my memory. The lady who escorted me to the door handed me her card. "Sweetie, just contact me if you need your records. And have a nice day."

Yeah right, I thought. *I'm going to throw this card away at the nearest trash can.*

When I got home, Bob and our daughter Meridith peppered me with questions. I couldn't answer. I was shaking. They had gotten me my favorite taco salad for supper, but I couldn't eat anything. I suddenly had no appetite and felt I would choke if I even tried to swallow. For months I couldn't talk about this traumatizing experience, not even with my family.

The Meeting

I could tell something was wrong—perhaps majorly wrong with my body. The doctors were not direct, but rushed and mysterious. Meanwhile, my anxiety was building. I needed some answers, and then I remembered that I might be able to contact a breast specialist.

When Bob first found the suspicious lump in January, I had contacted Mayo Clinic for a second opinion. They scheduled an appointment for me with a breast specialist. When my tests came back negative, however, I decided to cancel that appointment. I was glad to have the awareness, though, that breast specialists exist. Haunted by my recent experience at my local hospital, I asked my PCP if she could find me a breast specialist. She referred me to a breast specialist at a university hospital in our area, a hospital with the distinction of being a National Cancer Institute (NCI) Designated Cancer Center.

After my "bad" doctor appointment Bob and Meridith decided they would not let me be alone.

The three of us would be Siamese triplets; we were going to go everywhere together. What a comfort to know I didn't have to face this scary nightmare by myself. The NCI Center was a breath of fresh air! Manicured garden areas and blooming flower pots made a cheery entrance into big airy waiting rooms, often with many windows. We were greeted upon walking into each reception area and kindly directed to our destination. Beautiful artwork predominantly placed about dimmed the typical bland hospital walls that can scream "sick and dying." The medical professionals looked us in the eye, called me by name, welcomed all three of us with introductions and handshakes. Knowing this hospital had the latest technology and up-to-date research gave me confidence with their care.

Second opinions are fine, even necessary sometimes. Don't worry about offending your physician if you want to confirm your diagnosis with another medical professional or change to a different facility (or provider) you are more comfortable with. In fact, I had doctors who even suggested I check elsewhere before consenting to a treatment plan.

> ♛ *Second opinions are fine, even necessary sometimes. Don't worry about offending your physician.*

The breast specialist and her physician's assistant, introduced themselves warmly to each of us. They were appreciative that Bob and Meridith had both accompanied me, including all three of us in the discussion. The doctor's mannerisms had a calming effect, she appeared confident in her medical knowledge of breast cancer yet mirrored that with a desire to understand my unique situation. Everything the breast specialist and her PA did was "Like a gentle, cool rain shower on a stifling hot afternoon," as Meridith put it.

Compiling a thorough history on me, she rattled off one question after another on topics, ranging from breastfeeding to eating habits; from lifestyle to number of pregnancies; from exercise habits to overall health. The doctor and her PA also spent time listening to our concerns and answering any questions we had. We never felt insignificant or rushed. The doctor focused on risk factors that could lead to breast cancer: not being physically active, being overweight, taking oral contraceptives or hormone replacement therapy, having first pregnancy after age 30, never having a full-term pregnancy, not breastfeeding, drinking alcohol, being over 50, genetic mutations, menstrual periods before 12, menopause after 55, dense breasts, prior breast cancer, family history of breast or ovarian cancer, and previous radiation therapy. Amazingly, I hardly had any of these risk factors!

I reflected on the months leading up to the discovery of my own lump. I remember I would randomly get jabbing pains in my breast. They say you can't feel breast cancer, but I had that pain consistently. One cancer sign I did not have is unexplained weight loss. In fact, I had actually gained weight in the weeks prior to my diagnosis. I've learned that everyone's experience and symptoms are unique. Even knowing the breast cancer signs doesn't fully prepare you for receiving a diagnosis like this.

The breast specialist finished up the appointment with a breast exam. When she first saw my diseased breast, she didn't act shocked, as if I were a freak show. The doctor then straightened up and with a calming smile said, "First things first, let's get some tests done."

A few days later we triplets headed to an area of the NCI Hospital that is devoted exclusively to women and breast health. Even though I had brought along my imaging results from the other hospital (October 2014, January 2015, and June 2015), this hospital wanted to get their own. They recommended that I get the 3D mammogram, since all my past mammograms had been 2D. The mammographer smiled, called my name, asked if she pronounced it correctly, then introduced herself to all of us. I told her I was extremely nervous and asked if Meridith (who had just graduated from nursing school) could go in with me for the mammogram. She said she couldn't allow that due to the potential residual radiation that could transfer to Meridith. But, after closing the door, the mammographer did offer me a hug to help calm my nerves before starting the test. After the mammogram was over, she brought Meridith into the room while she interpreted the images of my breasts.

Meridith *was* able to be in the room with me and hold my hand during my repeat sonogram. My new radiologist studied the films, then examined me, noting the thickened skin on my right breast and enlarged lymph nodes under my arm. A few minutes later he sat down with Bob, Meridith, and *fully-clothed* me. Then he looked me in the eye and gently stated, "It's highly likely this is cancer. The biopsy results will tell us for sure." This was the first time a medical professional said the word "cancer" to me. This direct and honest verbiage was welcome!

Meridith, who was also allowed to accompany me for the biopsies, described the events like this: "A startling snap, like the sound of a staple gun, pierced the air as the needle procured its sample. Snap! Snap! The worst was over. Specimens were extracted from Mom's right breast, the skin of the breast above the tumor, as well as one lymph node under the right arm."

Each needle core biopsy hurt like a shocking stab, but the gentleness of the staff made it endurable. Being offered warm blankets often during these tests were an additional comfort, like receiving an extra hug.

The Verdict

Two days later, the quiet morning was interrupted by the sound of my ringtone. It wasn't in my purse or pocket, mind you! I had become too terrorized to have it in my possession. Meridith, who was the keeper of my phone, noticed it was the hospital's number calling, so she answered. The nurse said they had the results of my biopsies and wanted us to come in to visit with the doctor. She mentioned an appointment opportunity that afternoon or one the next week. I opted for the later one, but Meridith wisely chose the sooner appointment. We triplets arrived and were ushered into the doctor's office. I sat between Bob and Meridith, feeling as though we were defendants anticipating a verdict.

The breast specialist came in, warmly greeted us, then asked if we could switch up our seating arrangement so that she could sit next to me. Once we were all in place, she leaned forward, placed her hand on mine, and began, "Your biopsy and imaging results show you have a breast cancer called invasive ductal carcinoma." She proceeded to explain what it all meant in layman's terms, drawing pictures to help with understanding.

I felt as though I was in a dream as I sat there hearing the news that I indeed had breast cancer. I vividly remember the layout of the room and seating arrangement, but I felt distant. I had a tissue in my hand, thinking I would surely cry if I got a breast cancer diagnosis, but no tears came. Meridith later told me that when the doctor first mentioned that I had breast cancer, it hit her like a harsh slap to the face. She said she then had to pull her thoughts back to the doctor's words so she could be sure to get the facts and details. It is helpful to have someone with you to take notes at doctor appointments to help with the information overload that can come with a medical diagnosis.

The doctor continued, "The tumor is grade 2, about 4.5 cm, and has spread to the surrounding skin and at least one lymph node. I am suggesting a combination of chemotherapy, surgery, and radiation. You will lose your hair. You will lose your breast. But it is curable."

> *Take someone with you to take notes at appointments to help with information overload.*

She then answered our questions and attempted to calm our fears. Her familiarity was so comforting, I felt as though I was talking with a dear girlfriend when I asked, "I have a haircut and highlights scheduled in a few days, should I keep that appointment knowing I will be losing my hair in a few weeks?"

"Yes, I think so," she answered. "If it were me I know that would help me feel normal and good about myself." So I went ahead with my scheduled cut and color and, even added a pink streak in my hair in honor of breast cancer awareness.

The verdict: Breast Cancer Stage 3b. I would lose my hair, I would lose a breast, but it was curable.

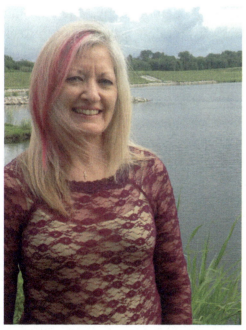

A few days after finding out I had breast cancer.

I couldn't help remembering Job's response to the tragic news of the death of his sons and daughters and the loss of all his earthly goods:

> Then Job arose and tore his robe and shaved his head, and he fell to the ground and worshiped.
>
> He said, "Naked I came from my mother's womb, and naked I shall return there. The LORD gave and the LORD has taken away. Blessed be the name of the LORD" (Job 1:20–21).

I bless Your name, God, even in this.

The Road Ahead

Five days after my diagnosis, we had my first appointment with my oncologist. "You will need eight rounds of chemotherapy," the oncologist explained, "one treatment every two weeks, totaling around sixteen weeks. I am recommending we begin next week." I sat with my faithful triplets in the little examination room, listening to the doctor and attempting to soak in the two-hour explanation of what to expect as treatment progressed, the myriad of side effects that could possibly occur with the chemotherapy drugs, and the battery of tests that would be needed prior to the first treatment: gene testing, blood tests, breast MRI, echocardiogram, positron emission tomography (PET) scan, and port placement for IV therapy. I couldn't get over how fast the information kept coming, how immediately I was getting appointments with these new doctors, how soon they scheduled my additional tests, and how quickly my active treatment would start.

I Have Cancer?

"It's everyone's greatest fear," a friend said.

"Really?" I replied. "I've never been afraid of getting cancer."

But, *after* I'd been diagnosed with breast cancer, I *was* scared! I selfishly remarked, "I don't want cancer." I prayed there would be another explanation to the growth in my breast. I told Bob, "I'm not afraid to die."

"Then don't be afraid to live," he quickly answered. I knew he was right. His admonition caused me to want to adjust my attitude, but this wasn't going to be easy. Choosing to live was a conscious choice that I had to make over and over throughout the ordeal.

Bob showed this act of living in this letter he wrote post-cancer diagnosis:

Camilla,

> "God is a very present help in trouble. But He permits trouble to pursue us, as though He were indifferent to its overwhelming pressure, that we may be brought to the end of ourselves, and led to discover the treasure of darkness, the unmeasurable gains of tribulation."
> – p. 26 of *Streams in the Desert* by Mrs. Charles E. Cowman

I love you, and I will be by your side no matter the path. We will face your fears together in the strength of our Lord and Savior, Jesus Christ—through whom we can do all things, all things, including the possibility of cancer.

–Bob

June 15, 2015 is the official date of my breast cancer diagnosis. That was also the date that one of my heroes of the faith and favorite radio teachers, Elisabeth Elliot, died. She would always start her daily radio program this way: "You are loved with an everlasting love. That's what the Bible says. And underneath are the everlasting arms. This is your friend, Elisabeth Elliot." Elisabeth ended her life with dementia. Some say she handled her death just as she did the deaths of her husbands—she accepted what came her way, knowing it was no surprise to God. She would rather not have experienced it, but she *received* it. I saw snippets of God's faithfulness in Elisabeth's life. And that gave me courage to trust that I would see snippets of His faithfulness in mine too.

This isn't the script I had written for my life. I hadn't planned on being interrupted with breast cancer, but this was now the path I was on. Our Pastor often says, "This didn't take God by surprise." That is true.

Regardless of what caused this cancer to grow in my breast, whether this came about because of something I did or didn't do, God still knew it was going to happen. He is omniscient. What if this was His plan for me all along? I need to realize that God is writing my story and I just need to hang on for the ride. After all, this was way more adventurous than what *I* would have written.

I remember in a weak moment many years ago, I agreed to jump on the back of a friend's motorcycle for a short ride. Now, *that* was wild for me! When he made his first right turn, and the motorcycle leaned right, I leaned left. Next, he and the motorcycle turned left, but I leaned hard right. He hollered back at me over the roar, "You have to lean with the motorcycle, otherwise we could wreck!"

Maybe now I needed to lean into God and trust Him on this new journey even if my tendency was to go the other way—even if it meant losing what I thought was my best feature.

CHAPTER 2

The Mom Becomes the Child

I Feel Like I Have Lost Control of My Life

I am an organized person. I use my Franklin Planner religiously, recording not only my appointments, but also what time I need to leave the house. The spices in my cupboard are alphabetized. The Greek yogurt and Kombucha in our fridge are lined up according to expiration dates. I keep record of all correspondence and gifts sent and received on 3x5 cards in my address file.

I also organized a health regimen for my family. Early on in my marriage I researched nutrition. My kids called me the ultimate health nut. I made them drink plenty of pure water, take good vitamins, eat lots of fruits, vegetables, and freshly ground grains. I even made them eat tofu and legumes regularly! Daily exercise, fresh air, and sunshine were also enforced. *Mean mom!* As for me, I kept regular well-woman checkups, never missed a mammogram, and followed the breast health guidelines—all recorded in my Franklin Planner, of course.

I had my life under control, but I still got cancer. After all of that—after abstaining from tobacco, keeping all my appointments, infusing my body with vitamins and whole foods . . . *cancer*!

After my diagnosis and my initial emotional breakdown, I was reminded that we don't have as much control as we think we do—if any! Even those of us who "take control" with planners and diet. This is the way Proverbs 16:9 puts it: "The mind of man plans his way, but the LORD directs his steps." God wants us to be wise and thoughtful and plan well, but we need to remember that He is ultimately in control. He is God, and we are not.

> *I had my life under control, but I still got cancer.*

This was not the first time I have had my plans crushed. Since my earliest memory, I had always wanted to be a wife and a mommy. I went to college right out of high school and graduated with a degree in Health Care Administration four years later. Shortly afterwards, I married my first husband. Eight months after we said, "I do," he left me and never returned—saying he decided he didn't love me after all. My dream was shattered.

During this dark and lonely time in my life as I dealt with this marriage crisis, God became my companion, and the Bible was my food. One morning I stumbled upon Psalm 37:4, which says, "Delight yourself in the LORD; and He will give you the desires of your heart."

Well, that can't happen to me now, I thought sarcastically! *How can I ever be a wife or mother without a husband?!* Then, I realized that if I truly make God my delight and focus on Him, He would take care of my desires (either by providing a husband and/or child, *or* by changing my desires so that I *longed* to be single). My job was to live my life for Him; the rest was in His very capable hands.

Two years later I met Captain Robert Crank on a blind date. Four months after we met, we were married, and I became a stay-at-home wife. When our first child, Thomas, was born, I was overwhelmed with gratitude that God had made me a mommy after all! God later blessed us with Kevin and then Meridith. I had the honor and privilege of nurturing and raising our precious children. I have enjoyed each stage of mothering, from babyhood through teenage years. Now I so appreciate seeing them each as responsible, God-fearing adults. I could truly agree with Psalm 107:1: "Oh give thanks to the LORD, for He is good, for His lovingkindness is everlasting."

Now that I faced another life crisis that threatened to confound my plans and dreams, I began to lean back into Psalm 37:4 and Psalm 107:1. The kindness of the Lord was indeed evident in the providential timing of my cancer diagnosis. Meridith graduated with her Bachelor's of Science in Nursing on May 10, 2015. She moved back home where she studied for and then passed the National Council Licensure Examination (NCLEX) on June 10th. Her first nursing job at The Mayo Clinic didn't begin until July. That meant that she was with us during each step down my unknown path of unexpected doctor appointments, tests, cancer diagnosis, and early treatments. Meridith headed up my medical responsibilities like an authoritative mom; I became a timid worried child trying my best to follow her directives. The security of Meridith's hugs calmed my troubled body! After all those years dispelling her fears with my enveloping hugs, now here I was on the receiving end. I had no idea the peace, comfort, and protection I would feel with a simple embrace from one of my offspring.

Not only was I now needing care, but I was in need of encouragement too. I am usually the encourager, the one reminding others of Psalm 37:4 or other truths about God's sovereignty, but this cancer diagnosis had derailed my well-laid plans, causing my feelings of confidence to melt into fear and helplessness. Now I had to *walk* the faith I so eagerly *talked* about.

Treatment Plan

My cancer team recommended chemotherapy before surgery because my cancer was fast-growing, so they wanted a systemic method that would treat the whole body first, allowing them to measure how effective the chemo was at shrinking the tumor. Additionally, my oncologist conducted a physical exam of my breast at every appointment to monitor the size of the lump.

After my chemotherapy treatment was complete, I would have a mastectomy, followed by thirty rounds of radiation, and then to top it all off I would take hormonal therapy pills for at least the next five years.

I was impressed at how my medical team educated us. These informational sessions often lasted at least an hour, and we felt like college students attending valuable lectures. My doctors never seemed rushed. At the end of detailed explanations, they would ask if we had questions and explain things in another way, if necessary. We were spoken to with compassion; we felt they were personally treating *me*, not just my disease. I received many personalized books with details of my type of cancer and specific treatment. These books contained messages of hope from fellow breast cancer survivors, an overview of my breast cancer diagnosis, details of my treatment plan, information about my medical team and facilities, and a glossary of common cancer terms. I referred to these resources often.

If I found myself confused about the medical information (as I often did), Meridith, would clarify. One time I was stumped when I saw that the oncologist's nurse practitioner (NP) gave me a prescription for a "cranial prosthesis." For a minute I wondered if I also had brain cancer, but Meridith told me this was just the medical way to say wig! We got some good laughs out of that one. In addition to the prescription, the NP presented a thorough explanation of the side effects of each of the chemotherapy drugs, steroid, white blood cell boosting drug, and a few anti-nausea medications included in my regimen. Meridith made the comment that my medication list, which previously consisted of a hypothyroidism drug and a handful of natural vitamins, "seemed to explode into a mountain of meds from about every genre in a matter of minutes."

Arming ourselves with the chemo nutrition booklet and pamphlet on managing chemo side effects, we triplets departed the office, ready to face this menacing foe that loomed before us.

Preparing for Treatment

Before cancer, the only hospitalizations I ever had was delivering our three children—and all without pain meds! I've even gotten fillings at the dentist without Novocain. I hadn't had any broken bones or surgeries. The only anesthesia I'd had was for my colonoscopy when I turned fifty! Now I was about to undergo the first surgery of my life! I was getting a Power Port inserted less than two weeks after discovering I had cancer.

My oncologist said I needed a port; otherwise, the chemo drugs he prescribed for me could destroy my veins. Also, the chemo mixes better in the blood with a Power Port because the port delivers it into a large central vein. My Power Port was a small device about the size of a quarter; it was placed under the skin on my left upper chest. The port had a small basin that was sealed with a soft silicone top called a septum. A catheter (tube) from the port was placed inside one of the large central veins that takes blood to the heart. Not only could chemotherapy, other medicine, and blood products be given through the needle, but also blood samples could be drawn from there, and it could be used for contrast injections for CT scans.

One week after first meeting my oncologist I changed into the customary hospital gown and climbed up on a gurney—two things that were new to me but would become very commonplace in the next few years. I was so comforted that Meridith was allowed to be there for all my pre-procedure prep. The RN showed us a model of the port and demonstrated how the infusion nurses would insert the needle to administer the chemo drugs. I was hooked up to an IV, blood pressure, and heart monitoring devices. "Keep your right arm straight, so the antibiotic can infuse," Meridith reminded me. "Now relax your left arm so the machine can take an accurate blood pressure."

Next thing I knew, they put a blue surgical cap on my freshly colored hair and wheeled me in for the first surgery of my life! My greatest fear in this first surgery (which the medical personnel kept telling me was really just a "procedure") was the anesthesia. I feared the idea of being in an unconscious state, totally unaware of what's going on, and not having control over my thoughts or actions. It was all an eerie feeling to me. It's weird I felt this way, as I don't have a fear of dying. They used conscious sedation, which is a mild form of anesthesia, and I didn't have any ill side effects from it.

Upon being released from the hospital, we triplets stopped off for a fun lunch with the rest of the family before heading home. I was feeling fine until the surgery pain meds wore off in the middle of the night. The pain got so intense I couldn't sleep. Meridith had given me a bell to ring in case I needed her in the night. Apparently, she was sleeping too soundly to hear my ringing, so I went into her bedroom. She woke up with a start and went into full nurse mode! She looked over my incision for possible infection or allergic reaction to the port material, checked for hemorrhaging, blood clot, asked about dizziness, shortness of breath, or fatigue. After I passed her assessment, we decided I would take some Tylenol (acetaminophen) then try Advil (ibuprofen) in the morning if the pain persisted.

The port insertion incisions healed and most pain subsided in about a week. After that point, there wasn't any extra port maintenance on my part. My port was painful, being a foreign object to my body, and it hurt a whole lot more with even the slightest bump. Car seatbelts were especially annoying as they pressed against the port. I decided to try using a soft infant seatbelt wrap to add a layer of cushion. Though I appreciated that relief, the symbolic nature of my daughter in the driver's seat and I with a child's car seat apparatus was not lost on me.

So It Begins

July 1st was Meridith's 22nd birthday, but instead of a big celebration, she was accompanying me to my first PET scan. I was very apprehensive about this scan as it would show if cancer had spread to other organs in my body. I was once again relieved they allowed Mom-Meridith into the prep room where they started an IV and injected my body with dye. After this, though, Meridith had to leave the now dark room lest she overstimulate me. I was told to lie still to allow the dye to spread through my body. I wasn't even allowed to read a book as any stimulus could cause the dye to congregate too much in one area. Meridith later reflected, "Looking back, I don't think I've ever been able to spend so much time with Mom as I

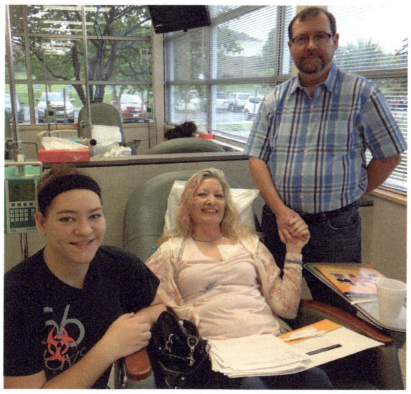

My first chemo.

have in the last few weeks. That's what has made this birthday so special; I got to spend quality time with my mother and give back to her what she has given me for twenty-two years."

Thursday, July 2nd was the scheduled day of my first chemotherapy. Of course, I had Bob and my Mom-Meridith by my side. First my blood was drawn from my freshly placed port; it just felt like a little pin prick when they inserted the special needle through the skin into the port.

Then we had an appointment with my oncologist. We were having trouble focusing on the lab numbers he was giving us, as our minds were wondering about the results of my PET scan, which would reveal if my cancer had spread to my uterus or ovaries. The doctor stopped mid-sentence when he noticed the anxious looks on our faces. "Let me put you at ease," he said. "The cancer has not spread to any other organs." Our sighs of relief were audible. We could breathe easily again. Only we still had one big hurdle: round one of chemotherapy.

Entering the infusion room felt surreal; I couldn't believe that I actually had breast cancer and was getting chemotherapy. The nurses gave me a quick tour of the room. There was a refrigerator for our use filled with Ensure, juices, and other snacks. There was a small library of books and games and a table with puzzles already in progress. They had me choose a recliner. I chose one close to the windows, as I wanted to look out to the well-manicured garden. The RN brought me a pillow and warm blanket, welcomed Bob and Meridith, and then once I got comfortable, she accessed my port. First, I was given a few IV anti-nausea medications and a couple of steroid tablets. Then it was time for the actual chemotherapy drugs. The nurses were very personable, talking and asking questions as they administered the drugs. Over my many hours spent in the infusion therapy room, it was clear that these nurses truly were interested in each patient's story.

My first chemo drug, Adriamycin (doxorubicin), was red. They had me eat a popsicle while it was infusing in hopes of preventing or reducing mouth sores. Research shows that chewing on cold items constrict the vessels in the mouth, which reduces the amount of blood containing the drug from reaching there. The second drug, Cytoxan (cyclophosphamide), was clear, but had a kick to it, causing increased sinus pressure and sneezing.

After my first chemotherapy treatment I was surprised that the effects didn't make me feel as bad as I thought they would! I went straight home, grabbed some things to read and a bucket—because, surely, I was going to throw up! I made a comfy spot on the sofa to recline and prepared for the worst. After an hour I felt fine, so I got up and did some housecleaning!

I was given strict orders to take anti-nausea medication at the first indication of nausea, but I have never been one to pop pills at every abnormal symptom. Later that afternoon, Meridith and Bob kept hounding me, ensuring I was following the doctor's orders. Feeling weak in the early evening, I surrendered again to the sofa. When they inquired if I was feeling nauseous, I stated, "Oh, it's not nausea, it's *pre-nausea*." Before the night ended, though, I submitted to my nagging family members and took the prescribed drug.

My chemotherapy infusion appointments would often take all morning. Family members always accompanied me, which made me feel like a well loved and cared for dependent. I would take books to read, my iPad, needle work, water, and something for us to eat. I did try to drink an Ensure, to boost my nutrients; I found it was more tolerable if I froze it for a short while to make it like a milkshake.

The treatment plan was four rounds of Adriamycin, which interferes with the growth and spread of cancer cells, along with Cytoxan, which slows or stops the growth of cancer cells. These infusions would be spaced two weeks apart. I would get a Neulesta (pegfilgrastim) shot to boost my white blood cells the day after receiving the treatments. This injection worked wonders in keeping up my white blood counts.

To make sure counts were high enough for another dose of the poison, I had blood work done immediately prior to each chemotherapy infusion. There was always the chance of postponing chemo for a week if my blood counts were too low, or I was considered too sick.

Though my chemo appointments were done every two weeks, I still had to report to the treatment center for blood work on each off week for the medical personnel to keep a close eye on my levels. It was like I had a standing appointment at this office every Thursday.

Adriamycin can cause cardio (heart) toxicity, so prior to my first chemo, I needed an echocardiogram (somewhat like a sonogram of the heart) to make sure my heart was healthy enough to take on the strain of chemotherapy.

Although I had been warned that the chemo drug Adriamycin can temporally cause red urine, it still came as quite a shock when it happened! I was still at the infusion center during my first chemo when this first happened to me. I thought, *Oh no! I need to tell the RN I'm bleeding!* Then I remembered the side effect warning. Also, Cytoxan can cause blood in the urine, so I was told to drink lots of water during the weeks I was receiving that chemotherapy.

The last of my chemotherapy drugs was four rounds of Taxol (paclitaxel), which prevents cancer cells from dividing; this was also administered two weeks apart.

I was prescribed Zofran (ondansetron) and Compazine (prochlorperazine) for nausea. Compazine is an antipsychotic, which is also used to treat anxiety and schizophrenia! One side effect is that the medicine can cause muscle movements that cannot be controlled, "tongue sticking out, puffing of cheeks, mouth puckering." A friend of mine said, "Will you please call me if that happens; I want to see what you look like!"

I also had to take Decadron (dexamethasone), a steroid, on days two, three, and four of each chemo cycle. This drug was great at keeping the nausea away, but, unfortunately, it would also keep the sleep away! I would routinely be awake 2–4 hours each night. I found having books on my iPhone handy as I could read while lying there in bed without turning on a light or causing much disruption for Bob.

I took Vitamin B6 to deal with temporary neuropathy (numbness) in my hands and feet that came with Taxol. I did have this syndrome for a few months. It was annoying, but not painful.

During the sixteen weeks of chemotherapy, they occasionally had me on Augmentin (amoxicillin) or Levaquin (levofloxacin) to fight infections. Meridith came up with the great idea for me to keep a running list of medications with the day and time they were to be taken. She then had me log the time I actually took each and the amount. This way she was assured that I was taking each medication as it was prescribed. Otherwise, with so many medications to keep up with over the course of treatment, it was easy to get confused. This drill reminded me of helping her organize her school assignments when she first started junior high.

I had two instances during chemotherapy treatment when I really thought I was going to throw up. I immediately took one of my anti-nausea meds, laid back in bed, and felt fine in fifteen minutes. It seems like medical chemists have gotten the drug concoction to attack chemo symptoms down to a science. I heard many fellow chemo patients talk about the absence of side effects and joking, "Are you sure you're really giving me chemotherapy, as I'm feeling fine?"

My oncologist said I would be fatigued about three to four days after each chemotherapy treatment, and yes, those were my hardest days in the cycle. I would be so fatigued that I couldn't stand for long, felt nauseous, and was weak. I reminded myself of my former adolescent kids so easily grumbling and complaining when not feeling well. It was a role reversal for me—my daughter being the leader and me the follower. Meridith had taken the reins, she was in charge. It was such a comfort, though, to rely on her to carry the load, help make decisions, give love and assurance when I was afraid.

On this unwanted journey, I found my spouse and children absolutely necessary to guide me and help me make decisions. I definitely needed to lean on them as they lived out Galatians 6:2: "Bear one another's burdens, and thereby fulfill the law of Christ." My breast cancer diagnosis was so overwhelming to me that it was not only *nice* for them to take the wheel, but I really *needed* them to get in the driver's seat. When our kids are young, we have the responsibility to make wise and loving decisions for them. As they grow, we help guide them as they learn to navigate life on their own. Then when we parents age, it is only natural that the tables are turned and our children are advising us. It reminds me of the brevity of humanity, the circle of life. What peace God provided me through my children! Looking back many years later I see the magnitude of how God really did give me the desires of my heart.

CHAPTER 3
God is Good

Am I Being a Baby About My Hair?

I love long hair—I've worn mine long most all my life, trying out many different styles when I was younger. My hair was a gift God gave to me, and I enjoyed it. As an adult, I let my hair stylist of twenty years experiment a bit with my style and color, but I had always kept the length! When I turned fifty, I asked her if I was too old for long hair. She said she'd let me know when the time came. Funny! I guess now the time had come!

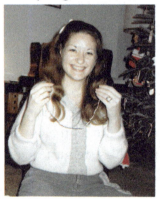 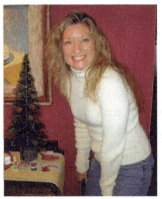 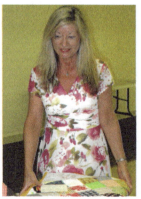

My hair through the years (from left to right): 80's, 90's, and 2010 when I was 50.

My hair started falling out profusely at our family reunion, about three weeks after my first chemotherapy treatment (just as the infusion RNs had predicted). In horror, I watched as my gift from God crumbled off my head and piled around me. What I didn't realize until later was that my balding was actually *part* of the gift.

I discovered that God is good, even in the bad. For example, even though I felt loss when Mom-Meridith moved out of state to start her nursing career, I felt great joy in seeing her accomplish her dream in working at the Mayo Clinic. She felt uneasy about leaving me, as I relied upon her so much that first month of my cancer diagnosis and treatment, but by the time she left, I was adjusting to my life of frequent doctor appointments and medical issues. I was ready to fully step into this next chapter of my life God was writing. It was time for her to start her career, and I still had Bob by my side. Fortunately, he was able to be with me at almost all appointments and treatments.

God Used the Babylonians

As Bob and I sat in the infusion room to receive my second round of chemotherapy I found it strange to think that I was purposefully allowing poisonous chemicals to be pumped into my veins, knowing it would destroy my cells. I voluntarily signed a written consent form agreeing to admit this killer into my blood to do its dirty work of destruction and death. This was necessary, though, to eliminate the cancer.

Scripture reveals that God can use the enemy in His work. As expressed in Habakkuk, God used the Babylonians (an evil people) to accomplish His will. God's purpose was to bring judgment on His own people for their idolatry. Babylon was the instrument of His judgment:

> "Look among the nations! Observe!
> Be astonished! Wonder!
> Because I am doing something in your days—
> You would not believe if you were told.

> "For behold, I am raising up the Chaldeans,
> That fierce and impetuous people
> Who march throughout the earth
> To seize dwelling places which are not theirs.
> They are dreaded and feared;
> Their justice and authority originate with themselves."
> ...
> Are You not from everlasting,
> O LORD, my God, my Holy One?
> We will not die. You, O LORD, have appointed them to judge;
> And You, O Rock, have established them to correct.
> – Habakkuk 1:5–7, 12

Similarly, unless the cancer patient knows why and how chemotherapy works, she could think the doctor was doing an evil thing to her. But this treatment is what is required, and it is necessary to save the patient.

We may struggle with questions about God's methods as Habakkuk did. Our wise and perfect God can, and sometimes does, use the sin already existing in our world to fulfill His purpose. Like Habakkuk, if we view life from God's perspective, our response will be to worship the Lord, knowing He is in control of all things. And this perspective allows us to worship even in the midst of absolute tragedy. Consider Habakkuk 3:17-19:

> Though the fig tree should not blossom
> And there be no fruit on the vines,
> Though the yield of the olive should fail
> And the fields produce no food,
> Though the flock should be cut off from the fold
> And there be no cattle in the stalls,
> Yet I will exult in the LORD,
> I will rejoice in the God of my salvation.
> The Lord God is my strength,
> And He has made my feet like hinds' feet,

And makes me walk on high places.

Sometimes the reason God doesn't change our situation is because He is trying to change our heart. Often, blessings begin with devastating circumstances.

> 👑 *Sometimes the reason God doesn't change our situation is because He is trying to change our heart.*

This lesson began to get clearer for me when my hair started coming out, my beautiful, long hair, my crown. As I said, it began to happen at our family reunion, and I could see God's hand even in this because we had taken a group photo on Friday night—the last night with my hair. What sweet timing!

The next morning in the shower my hair was coming out by the handful. I tried blow drying it, but now my hair was all over the sink, floor, and stuck to the walls. I kept scooping it up and putting it in the trash can until the waste basket was full. I warned the hotel maid, as I thought she'd think I had killed someone and stuck their head in the trash!

After returning home, my oldest son, daughter-in-law, and grandson came over to shave off what was left. One fear of mine was that I would scare my sweet grandbaby with my bald

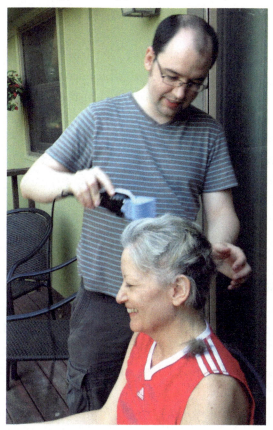
My son Thomas shaving my head.

head! Not to worry, he just sat witnessing the event then gave me a huge smile when it was all over!

Before my hair fell out, I had bought a wig, trying to pick something that looked as close as possible to my current hairstyle so no one would be able to tell I was bald! I bought a long straight blonde wig, thinking that would help me feel normal. Turns out, it was ridiculous! I only wore it out in public twice and felt unnatural both times.

I thought if I wore a wig I wouldn't stand out in the crowd. I found, though, that there are many people going through medical treatments nowadays that cause baldness. Also, shaved heads appear to be in style, and hats are popular. It was no big deal to be bald in public. I never once felt like a spectacle.

I was actually most comfortable with just a soft hat. I bought a few head coverings myself, but most were given to me as gifts. Some hats were even hand made. I had something to match every outfit. I also tied scarves around my head and even learned how to make cool head coverings out of old t-shirts. I occasionally went bare-headed at home, but not often, as I was bald during fall and winter, which made for a cold head if left uncovered. Upon advice received from a cancer survivor, I sewed myself a satin pillowcase as that was soothing to my bald head.

One new perk from this hair-loss side effect was that I no longer needed to shave my legs. In fact, I no longer had *any* body hair, including no eyebrows, eyelashes, or pesky facial hairs to pluck. It's an unusual sensation. It definitely makes showering faster! The time it took me to get ready in the morning was cut in half, since I no longer had the long hair to wash, dry, and style. I found that baby shampoo was the most soothing and all that was needed. The loss of eyebrows and eyelashes sometimes resulted in getting specks in my eyes. And, I lost my nose hairs, which meant a constant, annoying, drippy nose.

It was a very difficult thing for me to lose my hair. I felt I lost my femininity and looked unattractive with my bald head! But, when looking in the mirror and not happy with the reflection staring back at me, I found if I smiled my reflection looked much better. The best accessory I could put on each day was a smile.

As I look back over my cancer journey, I find so many ways God was good, but His perfect timing truly stands out. New medical professional appointments and tests continued to fill my calendar. We scheduled my breast reconstruction surgery shortly after I met my plastic surgeon in order to get a place in his busy schedule. We estimated the date to fit six weeks after the conclusion of my cancer treatment. Meridith asked off work and booked flights home many months in advance in order to be with me in the hospital and recovery. Our military son wanted to fly home to see me before my surgery, but he didn't have control of his availability. I often prayed about the parts of this puzzle and how they would all fit together. I couldn't be sick or surgery would have to be rescheduled, which would be nearly impossible for my plastic surgeon as this surgery takes a full day in the operating room. I kept watching and praying.

A few days before the surgery, the hospital called saying my insurance hadn't yet been approved, which could cause a delay. Then, my oncologist called with concerns about being off a particular medication a few weeks, another possible delay. I was nervous and getting cold feet about the whole procedure, wondering if I could go through with it. As the time drew nearer, I watched God cause all the pieces to fall into place, including our Navy son's visit just prior to surgery, everything was answered according to what was best and needed.

Though now I can clearly see how God was good, in the moment when I was waiting for answers to prayer and struggling with the unknowns, I wondered if He had forgotten about me. Would this really turn out for good?

When we're upset, we tend to pick up the phone and rant to a girlfriend. Psalm 55:17 gives us a better way to vent: "Evening and morning and at noon, I will complain and murmur, and He will hear my voice." God wants to be the first to hear our cares. I have grown accustomed to walking around my house, talking out loud to Him about all my frustrations. This doesn't offend God, in fact He invites our complaints.

In addition to talking with God in prayer, I found that the Bible provides answers when nothing else makes sense. In difficult times, we are drawn to His word for direction and help as Psalm 119:105 says, "Your word is a lamp to my feet and a light to my path." No other book can satisfy like the Bible. It is a living book that can decipher our thoughts as stated in Hebrews 4:12, "For the word of God is living and active and sharper than any two-edged sword, and piercing as far as the division of soul and spirit, of both joints and marrow, and able to judge the thoughts and intentions of the heart." It accomplishes a purpose according to Isaiah 55:11: "So will My word be which goes forth from My mouth; it will not return to Me empty, without accomplishing what I desire, and without succeeding in the matter for which I sent it." It contains all the wisdom we need to live on this earth as James 1:5 says, "But if any of you lacks wisdom, let him ask of God, who gives to all generously and without reproach, and it will be given to him."

Due to the distress of my cancer diagnosis, sometimes I couldn't stomach eating food. During those times, though, I could feast on the Word of God. It truly brought me comfort and provided direction. It redirected my focus on God's goodness. God is the One who made us, so, surely, He knows what we need or don't need. He is even better than we are at determining our wants and desires. Consider Jesus' response to Satan in Matthew 4:4 when he was famished after he hadn't eaten for forty days, But He answered and said, "It is written, 'Man shall not live on bread alone, but on every word that proceeds out of the mouth of God.'"

Reading the Bible brought me such comfort, I knew that memorizing portions of it would be a great help to me as well. Memorizing scripture is hard work! I find it laborious and easy to neglect. But, in difficulties, memorizing the Bible brings peace. Psalm 119:165 says, "Those who love Your law have great peace, and nothing causes them to stumble." I decided to keep my memory verses in a holder on the kitchen table and practice them daily before breakfast and lunch (I have included a list of some of my favorite scripture memory verses in Appendix B). The memorized verses naturally come to mind and are a reliable guide for living. I knew of a missionary couple, Martin and Gracia Burnham, who were abducted with only the clothes on their backs and held captive for over a year in the Philippine jungles. They would quote previously-memorized Bible verses to each other daily. This was their only "Bible" until they were released.[1] How many verses would I be able to recall if this happened to me? This challenged me to memorize more.

> ♛ *I kept my memory verses in a holder on the kitchen table and practiced them daily before breakfast and lunch.*

Richer

It's strange to say this, but cancer made my life richer. I learned to let go of the things that really weren't so important and began to focus my life on what mattered for eternity.

I woke up with joy more often, realizing that each day was a gift from God. We already know this, but seldom act on it.

My days became more fulfilling as I enjoyed the people God brought into my life. I began to see them as blessings, not burdens.

I even developed a different attitude concerning errands. Before getting cancer, I would be more focused on getting them done, getting home, then doing the next thing. After cancer, I realized that God could be using me in those insignificant encounters with strangers to bless someone's day. Sometimes all it takes is a smile, other times it might be paying for groceries, or an offering of prayer.

What I had previously thought were interruptions were often God's redirection for my day and where true fulfillment was found.

There was suffering in my cancer trial, but I can honestly say there was also good in it.

A Bump in the Road

I was walking through life, taking care of my responsibilities, living the life I felt God called me to when BAM, I hit a bump in the road—I found out I had breast cancer.

I learned, though, that this bump actually could become a high point in my life! It drew me closer to the Lord—what could be higher than that?! The bump, caused by my lump, forced me to deeper faith. I prayed earnestly, crying out to God Almighty, often with sweat and tears, as He is the One who could truly help me. I read the Bible more, as it was the only book that fulfilled my longings. And I memorized life-giving scriptures, as my mind wandered on unpleasant thoughts if I didn't continually remind myself of the truth.

When faced with a crisis in our lives, we are often at the end of ourselves—we need God's power (as if we didn't need it before!). Telling God my concerns and watching for His provision is a faith builder for me. Psalm 5:3 says, "In the morning, O LORD, You will hear my voice; in the morning I will order my prayer to You and eagerly watch."

Before I knew it, all of that praying, Bible reading, and verse learning turned this cancer bump in the road into a mountain-top experience. In even the most difficult circumstances, God provides peace and joy when we draw near to Him. I guess I'm making mountains out of molehills!

CHAPTER 4

Family and Such

od made us relational; we need each other. This is especially true when going through difficulties.

Sisters

My sisters were invaluable to me when I was dealing with my breast cancer diagnosis.

I, Camilla Adele, am the middle of five children.

Catherine Alice, our oldest sister, is a retired school teacher. Cynthia Arlene, second, was the Director of Health Services in a large school district. The youngest girl, Clarissa Ann, was formerly in the death care business. We also have a brother, Cary Allen, an elementary school principal, but this section is about sisters.

It turns out that Clarissa, my little sister (as I call her), and I had the most availability for several years, so we became Mom and Dad's assistants. Hence, we had many opportunities to take our parents to doctor procedures, talk on the phone, shop, and travel together.

In fact, she was my traveling buddy once again to help me with the move of Meridith's household goods. She left her home to drive seven hours to mine, so that we could then drive seven hours to Rochester, as my doctors didn't want me traveling alone.

After arriving at Meridith's new apartment, we immediately began cleaning so that we would be prepared to receive her shipment the next morning. Sure enough, the movers arrived as promised, first unloading the piano, which has been in my mom's family since the early 1900s. They continued swiftly carrying in boxes and the rest of the furniture for the next hour, asking Meridith where each item was to be placed and hollering off numbers for her to mark off her "bingo sheet." All the while, Clarissa and I steadily opened and unpacked the incoming boxes, continuing long after the movers left. We broke only for a quick walk, making dinner, and putting up beds so we could sleep. Meridith worked her shift at the hospital the next day, but that didn't deter Clarissa and me from continuing our attack of the boxes, paper, and clutter. We also became interior decorators. The four days we were together helping Meridith were my "best" days on my chemo calendar, something only God could orchestrate, and for that I am very thankful.

Soon Clarissa and I were back in the car for the return drive to my home. The next day she accompanied me to chemo round three. We were continually amazed at the positive outlook of the patients all around as they willingly shared their much more grim diagnoses than mine. They were looking on the bright side and enjoying life—getting better, not bitter. One patient with a rare form of brain cancer said he lost his peripheral eyesight. I feel like my sisters were acting as *my* peripheral vision. All three helped me see in this journey in the way they are each uniquely gifted.

I love my sisters and can feel their love for me, especially during this new road I'm traveling. Cathy has mailed me a plethora of encouraging cards with scriptures and called regularly to check on me. Cindy sent me chocolate covered strawberries early on when I was too nervous to eat much else. So paranoid, in fact, that when the phone call came concerning a delivery of "edible arrangements" I thought they were asking to make "medical arrangements!" Cindy also has been invaluable in translating medical jargon. Clarissa, Cindy, and Cathy, oh how I love you three!

Before Clarissa left for home, we attended a very informative seminar on breast reconstruction. With more options than I could have ever imagined, it was great to have an extra set of ears there with me! This was the perfect time in my cancer journey to hear this information, early enough to weigh all the options and do needed research, yet far enough in treatment to adequately understand the specific needs and limitations of my body.

Many possibilities were discussed, but the one I was most intrigued with was the Deep Inferior Epigastric Perforator (DIEP) flap reconstruction, which uses the tummy tissue to rebuild breasts. The updated part of this procedure is that the abdominal muscles aren't removed with the fat anymore. Instead the surgeon performs microsurgery, procuring tiny blood vessels with the tummy fat, then he reattaches the vessels to blood supply at the chest area.

We also were informed of 3D nipple and areola tattooing. Many women are choosing to forgo a new molded nipple, as they are always erect. Plus, the 3D tattoos are very realistic looking. Nipple sparing is available to some patients, but this doesn't guarantee nipple sensation. Also, preserved nipples could move to an awkward spot during reconstruction. I already knew that nipple sparing wasn't an option for me, as my tumor was directly under my nipple. I sure had a lot to think about as my sister Clarissa drove the seven hours back home.

Can We Talk About My Parents?

Of course, great sisters didn't just happen by chance. They were the result of a terrific upbringing.

My father, Guy Bill Stamps, was born the third of four boys to farming parents in Kingston, Arkansas. They were poor in the way of money, but rich in family love. Dad never left his hometown area until he went to School of the Ozarks for his senior year of high school. At this school the hard work ethic that had been instilled in him from birth continued, as he worked in the canning factory to pay for his schooling. Not long after graduating, he joined the United States Air Force. He soon got stationed at Wichita, Kansas.

There he looked up a cousin, who introduced him to her best friend, Rebecca Ann Ketteman, our future mom. Mom's father was a German master baker who came to America in 1923 for a few years to earn some money, then planned to return to his homeland. But while here, he met, fell in love, was married, and became a loyal American citizen. Mom was their middle child and only daughter. Mom's mother tragically died when Mom was at the tender age of thirteen. Grandmother Ketteman's belongings remained in the home as she left them, yet my Grandfather and their three children were to carry on without her. They lived on with broken hearts.

Guy and Rebecca were married August 7, 1954. They were blessed with a baby ten months later. Before long, they were parents of four daughters and one son. They made family their priority, and we became their hobby. Dad worked several jobs to provide for us. He also studied to earn his Bachelor's degree (double major in education and business). He then earned a Master's degree in education administration. In spite of losing her mom at an early age, our mom became the best mom in the world. She made the home her focus.

Of all the things my parents instilled in me, these five traits stuck with me the most:

> **(1) Service:** My whole life I have witnessed my parents lovingly care for many relatives, neighbors and friends. When they had Dad's mom and Mom's dad in the same nursing home, they visited twice a day, not only serving their own parents, but other residents as well. Now, they are always willing and able to help us with household projects, also helping their grandkids in their homes.

(2) **Hard Work:** I don't ever remember Dad or Mom complaining about the jobs they had to do at home or elsewhere; I just remember them working. And we children were expected to do the same. They still work at quilting, gardening, cashiering at their retirement complex's thrift store, baking pies and cookies for neighbors, and visiting shut-ins.

(3) **Consideration:** They are always thinking of others before themselves. Several years ago they bought a home in a retirement community, when they still felt too young to live there. They wanted to make this move before their children would need to make the decision for them. This complex also has apartments, assisted living, and skilled nursing care, in case they ever need more help. Additionally, in deciding on their burial spot, Dad and Mom's main concern was the convenience for us kids! They recently took us to see their fully-paid-for and erected tombstone. They have honored us by listing their five children's names on it.

(4) **Loyalty:** Mom and Dad have celebrated over sixty-five years of marriage. If they say they will do something, they will; they are faithful to keep their word. They will also always lend an ear to any child, grandchild, or great grandchild who needs someone to listen.

(5) **Generosity:** We gather as a family once a year; we children alternate hosting. Dad and Mom pay for the lodging for all of the out of town guests. They have helped furnish grandchildren's homes. They love to take any and all of the family out to eat.

Once when I had finished taking Mom and Dad to a doctor appointment, Mom said, "Thank you, until you are better paid." I then replied, "Mom, you have already paid in advance!"

How we five kids have been blessed!

And you know what? My elderly parents went with me to my fourth round of chemotherapy!

Brothers and Genes

My parents wanted a boy from their first pregnancy, even having his name picked out from the start—Cary Allen. When their first baby was a girl, they decided to use the same initials, hence Catherine Alice. Then came another girl, then another, then another. They decided the sure way to get a boy was to adopt! We were thrilled to get Cary when he was only one month, one week, and one day old. We loved that little guy from the very beginning and couldn't imagine our lives without him. He completed our family.

As he grew and would go to the doctor, we realized we had no medical history on him; we didn't share genes with him.

My oncologist strongly urged me to do the gene testing. He couldn't guarantee that it would be covered by insurance, but he felt the knowledge would be invaluable to my family. At many annual mammograms prior to my diagnosis, I had repeatedly been asked per written form if I desired genetic testing. I had always responded "yes"; however, this was the first time a medical person actually followed through with the request.

Blood work was all that was required from me, then it was sent to Myriad My Risk. Result: "negative—no clinically significant mutation identified". These are the genes that were analyzed: APC, ATM, BARD1, BMPR1A, BRCA1, BRCA2, BRIP1, CDH1, CDK4, CDKN24, CHEK2, EPCAM, MLH1, MSH2, MSH6, MUTYH, NBN, PALB2, PMS2, PTEN, RAD51C, RAD51D, SMAD4, STK11, and TP53. This was good news not only for me, but also for my sisters and children. However, I couldn't give any reassurance to my adopted brother.

I also am an adopted child, not in my physical family but in the family of God. Our family had always gone to church, so I thought I must have been born a Christian. I don't ever remember not believing in Jesus and God. A few times I even accepted Christ into my heart, while attending a crusade or watching a televangelist. I wanted that ticket to Heaven. It wasn't until my sophomore year in college, though, that I realized I needed to make a decision for Christ to be my *Lord* and not just my *Savior*. I needed to make Jesus the captain of my ship! I realized that if I accepted Him as my Lord and Savior, my life no longer belonged to me, but to Him.

Now that was something I could share with my sweet little brother. I loved him so much that I couldn't bear thinking of going to Heaven without him. The next time I was home from college, I remember explaining my new-found faith to him.

Friends

Being adopted into the family of God brings with it lots more brothers and sisters in Christ as stated in Ephesians 1:5, "He predestined us to adoption as sons through Jesus Christ to Himself, according to the kind intention of His will." These brothers and sisters provided help to me in so many ways.

As I pause to reflect on the events of my cancer diagnosis and treatment, I am reminded over and over again that I did not walk this trial alone. Here are just a few ways the body of Christ carried me and my family through the storm.

Our pastor and his wife came over immediately after my scary doctor appointment to comfort us and pray with us.

A friend organized an army of prayer warriors to pray for me every day—assigning a specific date to 31 different people who committed to pray for me on that date every month for one year.

Another friend went to all our neighbors to tell them about my diagnosis; I wanted them to know (in case they were frightened by seeing me bald), but I didn't want to be the one to tell them.

I was on church prayer lists all over the country; people who didn't even know me, including missionaries around the world, were praying for me.

I received over 400 encouraging cards, many with specific scriptures written in them and meaningful comments to meditate on.

Bob's workplace invited me to an in-person meeting to pray over me.

Neighbors, friends, and family brought countless meals regularly throughout the year, oftentimes just dropping off food or snacks unannounced.

I was showered with an array of presents, from hand knitted hats and homemade toiletries, to trinkets, scarves, and gift cards.

Upon entering church sporting my newly-grown-in-very-short hair style, friends cheered for me all the way from the front door to my seat. I felt like I was their favorite sports star running through a human tunnel to the court.

Even during routine errands, business workers gave me hugs and offered practical advice.

I had offers to clean our house, drive me to appointments, do my laundry, go out to eat, just visit, or take walks. People really were the hands and feet of Jesus to me and my family.

Family and friends have continued to serve me even months after my treatment ended when I still didn't feel up to par.

Sometimes I got some unusual advice. I had to learn how to graciously accept it, examine it, and decide whether to heed it or toss it out. Someone suggested I try pressing fresh pineapple onto the open wounds that chemo caused in my mouth. No thanks!

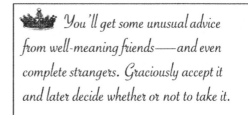
You'll get some unusual advice from well-meaning friends—and even complete strangers. Graciously accept it and later decide whether or not to take it.

Even the unusual advice is given in love.

Even the unusual advice was given in love—I could feel that. So much good advice can be overwhelming. I then had to rely on my family and God to figure out how we were going to treat this. I think this was another way my friends could help me fight.

What was most helpful was friends just *doing* things for us, rather than saying, "Call me if you need anything" or even, "What do you need?" As I ponder all my friends have done for me, I think they could write the book entitled *What to Do When Your Friend Gets Cancer*.

I couldn't have handled breast cancer without the people in my life. I have been blessed by an exceptional extended family and am extremely grateful for that. Maybe you look at your life and say you weren't so lucky in the way of family. But we can all have an unbelievably great family of God. God is the perfect heavenly Father and will heal us, teach us, help us, and always love us. He wants you in His family: "The Lord is not slow about His promise, as some count slowness, but is patient toward you, not wishing for any to perish but for all to come to repentance" (2 Peter 3:9).

One of my friends who was walking this cancer journey with me said, "I am praying that at least one person will come to know the Lord through your testimony." Maybe that person is you?

Romans 10:9–10 explains the way you can be in God's family: "... if you confess with your mouth Jesus as Lord, and believe in your heart that God raised Him from the dead, you will be saved; for with the heart a person believes, resulting in righteousness, and with the mouth he confesses, resulting in salvation."

Once in the family of God, it is essential that you find a good church home that preaches the Bible and then lives out what the Bible teaches. Our church was great at demonstrating Philippians 2:4: "do not merely look out for your own personal interests, but also for the interests of others." They helped us in innumerable ways. The body of Christ is supposed to be like this.

CHAPTER 5

Time Well Spent

Using the Blue Side

People often say, "God won't give you more that you can handle." But in reality, He *does* give us more than we can handle *so that* we will learn to lean on Him and not just rely on ourselves.

Some friends sewed me a pink infusion blanket with the breast cancer ribbon symbol quilted all over the top. Green used to be my favorite color, but I have embraced pink more since being diagnosed with breast cancer. They made the underside blue. "Turn it over whenever you feel blue," they said.

I turned it over and kept it blue side up for several weeks. This cancer journey was getting old, and at times I bordered on being depressed. I was getting tired of the side effects of chemo: aches, fatigue, insomnia, mouth sores, feeling puny. Sometimes it felt like my life was on hold. The world was continuing, and I was sitting on the sidelines. I was at the point where it had become an endurance test.

These feelings, I know, aren't unique to someone going through a crisis. We all go through mundane, boring, and low times in our lives. When my kids have expressed loneliness, I encourage them to go find another human to encourage. In so doing we find ourselves uplifted. My mom often says, "Keep on keeping on."

Dealing with cancer was like having a part-time job—so many appointments to go to and suffering through a myriad of side effects. Then the bills start coming, and all that paperwork is another part-time job.

I felt like I had lost myself somewhere and didn't know where to find me! It had been so long since I felt well. I didn't even know my name anymore. I've always gone by "Camy," but "Camilla" is on all my documentation. *Camilla* rhymes with Pamela, but every new medical person I met pronounced it differently. I'd sit in waiting rooms never knowing what name I would be called.

Also, chemotherapy had suddenly put my body into menopause, so I was dealing with frequent hot flashes, a fuzzy mind, sleep disturbances, and moodiness on top of everything else. Even though I was part-way through chemo, I still had surgery, radiation, reconstruction, and hormonal therapy to go; there was still a long road ahead! Cancer fighting was a marathon, not a sprint.

Next up I had a good visit with my breast surgeon. She was very pleased at how well the tumor was responding to the chemo. She could physically feel it had shrunk, which would make surgery easier.

Then I saw my plastic surgeon and my new PCP. They all seemed smart, well-educated, trustworthy, and very capable to care for me. But, goodness, I was getting tired of being examined, looked at, photographed, and poked! And so much information kept swirling around in my brain: double mastectomy, lymph node removal, tissue expanders, implants, DIEP flap reconstruction, and Liposuction Fat Transfer. I was apprehensive about the next step, mastectomy, but my breast surgeon said that this was the time to build up my strength. Do what makes me happy, and stay healthy!

God's encouragement to me from James 1:2–3 was, "Consider it all joy, my brethren, when you encounter various trials, knowing that the testing of your faith produces endurance." Our first inclination when a trial comes is to turn and run the other way. Growth comes, however, when we face the trial head on. This is how my pastor puts it: "The way you gain endurance is by enduring something." Many times, I felt like what I was going through was too much for me to bear. I was lacking endurance but found if I just took the first step then simply did the next thing, I continued to gain more than I started with. At the end of a specific difficult period, I could look back and see God's faithfulness, my growth, and feel joy from the fruit of my labor. This actually helped me have the courage to flip the quilt back over to the pink side.

Trudging Along

The effects of chemotherapy got progressively worse with each infusion. I became weaker and needed to rest more. Besides fatigue, I developed fever blisters on my lips, a sore throat, mouth sores, insomnia, and slight fevers. Pre-nausea was my constant companion.

Mouth sores were a painful, pesky annoyance. My doctor prescribed Magic Mouthwash (xyloxadryl), a numbing medicine that I could rinse with before eating. That proved frightening to me as it not only numbed my ability to feel the open sores, but it also hindered my ability to feel my mouth. I tried it while eating out with family, couldn't feel what I was chewing and swallowing, and therefore almost choked! I found myself dreading eating. This was a short-lived side effect, so I was able to temporarily cope with a liquid diet. I did discover that putting the numbing medicine on a q-tip, then applying it only to the sores was beneficial. Lemon drops were soothing too.

Whatever I was able to eat during my chemo phase of cancer treatment became nauseating to me later on. I decided to hold off on eating my favorite foods for a while, so they could still be a favorite after chemo.

As my chemotherapy treatments continued, I was also more prone to infections. My oncologist didn't want me taking vitamin C, as it could combat the chemo. I would drink lots of water, tea with lemon and honey, and diffuse essential oils.

All my chemotherapy treatments went on as scheduled. I was pleasantly surprised I was able to receive chemo number seven as I had spent most of the two weeks leading up to it with a sore throat, a cough, sneezing, a runny nose, and fatigue. If my blood work showed low white blood cell count (WBC), that meant my body was too busy fighting an infection to receive another round of chemotherapy, as chemo also lowered WBC. Chemo would then have to be delayed, which could cause the cancer to start growing again. In order to continue my road to healing, I really wanted to keep on schedule.

A few times we witnessed someone getting to ring the bell in the infusion room after they completed their last chemo treatment. It's believed that this tradition began at MD Anderson in 1996. A U.S. Navy rear admiral was undergoing cancer treatment. He told his oncologist that he planned to follow a Navy tradition of ringing a bell to signify "when the job was done." The admiral proceeded to bring a brass bell to his last treatment and rang it. This tradition caught on in many, if not most, cancer centers across our country. Everyone in the infusion room—cancer patients, family members, and medical personnel, stop what they are doing to celebrate with the chemotherapy graduate. I anticipated this would soon be me. It seemed like such an insignificant way to herald the huge hurdle just accomplished, but I appreciated the effort of the staff to bring jubilation into a grim situation.

Another scary side effect of chemotherapy I had was heart pounding, which happened when I climbed hills, stairs, or tried to speed walk. This eventually subsided.

Speaking of walking, it had become my happy place. I found I only felt "good" when I was actually walking, so I did it daily and had family and friends who would join me. It seemed as though all the drugs in my body could pull me down and make me feel like doing nothing. As soon as I tied my sneakers and headed outdoors, I began to feel better emotionally and physically. The fresh air felt good in my lungs. The exertion caused my heart to beat faster, making me feel more alive. Being outside took the focus off me, allowing an opportunity to worship the Almighty through His glorious creation.

Some friends suggested we register in the Race for the Cure. The race coincided with the "worst" days of my chemo cycle, but my friends assured me they would support me in any way necessary. They were right! They drove me there and catered to my every need. They surprised me with additional family and friends who walked with us in support through this journey. It was a thrilling day to be around so many breast cancer survivors. I wore a pink survivor shirt, not quite understanding the meaning. I guess, once we're diagnosed, we are a survivor until we die.

Human Doing

Chemotherapy hampered me to where I wasn't very productive. I felt incompetent and inadequate and couldn't do the things I used to do. When I tried, my results weren't up to par and that frustrated me. Then God reminded me that I am a human *being* not a human *doing*. Why, then, do I work so hard at doing things? Maybe I needed to spend more time *being* rather than *doing*. Be with God, be with family, be with friends, be present, be in the moment.

I needed to practice what Psalm 46:10 says, "Cease striving and know that I am God; I will be exalted among the nations, I will be exalted in the earth."

God, His word, and people—these are the three things I discovered should be my priority. Giving people our time is a priceless gift. Through the years I have had people say to me, "Thank you for sharing your time with me." Older people often say, "One thing I have is time" or "Time is all I've got." I find this ironic, since the older we get, the less time we actually have on this earth! I guess as we age, we finally realize how to use our time on the things that really matter.

My idea of how to spend time well changed. I had started off feeling like I was sitting on the sidelines and couldn't do much. But then I realized that I could spend time encouraging others through texts, phone calls, and especially prayer. None of that valuable time was wasted. Time spent with God in prayer, study of His word, and being with people is truly time well spent.

Olives

Between each different type of treatment (chemotherapy, mastectomy, radiation, reconstruction, and hormonal therapy), my doctors gave my body a four- to six-week break. This gave my system a chance to bounce back and gain some strength before getting attacked again.

I knew I needed that time in between treatments to recover from all my body had been going through. The time-off after my mastectomy happened to fall in the midst of the holiday season. Christmas is busy enough on its own, but I felt handicapped that year with my "chemo brain." My brain felt like a pinball machine. As I tried to think about something, my brain went off doing something else. Multi-step tasks were next to impossible—first plan meals, second check for ingredients, third make grocery list—I would go to the pantry to look for a necessary ingredient having to continually repeat it until I determined if the item needed adding to the list.

I had trouble focusing on "necessary" tasks we give ourselves this time of year. When asked to bring a food item for our first Christmas gathering, I simply chose to take olives. Then I decided to take olives to the next event, then the following one! Normally, I would have searched recipes and chosen the perfect dish to prepare for each occasion. But, that year it was just olives, and that was okay.

It reminded me of the story of Mary and Martha in Luke 10. In verses 41 and 42, Jesus says, "Martha, Martha, you are worried and bothered about so many things; but only one thing is necessary, for Mary has chosen the good part, which shall not be taken from her." It was necessary for me to remember the true reason of Christmas, celebrating the birth of Christ. So many of our preparations steal our time from the good part. That year I was forced to scale back. This gave me the opportunity to see the simplistic pure beauty in the Christmas story, and I never wanted to veer from that again.

A Red-Letter Day

When I was young and had a milestone moment in my life, Mom used to say, "This is a red-letter day." I woke up the morning of my last chemotherapy treatment thinking about that. Bob and I were wondering what the saying really meant, so we Googled it!—"any day of special significance, important day or memorable day." It refers to the old custom of printing holidays in red on the calendar.

Red letters remind me of Jesus' words, which are printed in red in my Bible. Some of those most important words and, probably most quoted words of the Bible are John 3:15–18: "so that whoever believes will in Him have eternal life. For God so loved the world, that He gave His only begotten Son, that whoever believes in Him shall not perish, but have eternal life. For God did not send the Son into the world to judge the world, but that the world might be saved through Him. He who believes in Him is not judged; he who does not believe has been judged already, because he has not believed in the name of the only begotten Son of God."

In facing my life-threatening disease, I found great comfort to have the assurance of salvation and a home in Heaven. This was possible for me not because of any good that I had *done*, but only

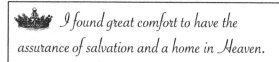
I found great comfort to have the assurance of salvation and a home in Heaven.

because I had *believed* in Christ as my Lord and Savior. I felt compelled to share this good news to those I encountered, especially to those staring death in the face. I felt drawn to the Bible, as its' words truly are life giving. I determined to pray for the salvation of the people I came across every day—*that*, if nothing else, made it time well spent.

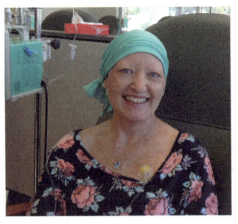
My last chemo treatment.

My final Chemotherapy was a red-letter day for me! I graduated and rang the bell! Even though I was still far from eradicating my cancer, it felt good to have finished this first phase. As Bob and I celebrated with a steak dinner, we reflected on God's faithfulness to us along this unchosen-by-us breast cancer journey.

CHAPTER 6

Removal

My bilateral mastectomy was scheduled for Wednesday, November 11, 2015. By God's perfect timing Meridith had already booked a flight to come home the previous weekend for her alma mater's homecoming so was then able to extend her stay to be my private nurse following my surgery. My blood work, chest X-ray, and EKG all checked out okay, so surgery was on.

I began packing a hospital bag and looking over all the pre-surgery instructions: which meds to stop and when, which meds to take, specific bathing soap and directions, fasting time, and so forth. I still had a few days before surgery, and I. Was. *Scared*. Thinking about getting my breasts cut off was a grotesque thought. Formerly when I had heard of someone getting breast cancer, I was horrified to think of them losing their breasts, a mark of womanhood. Now, here I was in that predicament. Waves of poignant memories of breastfeeding our three children and the pleasure my breasts brought during intimate times with my husband kept flooding my mind.

Meridith reminded me to rest in the Lord as I faced these fears. I turned to Psalm 56:3–4a, "When I am afraid, I will put my trust in You. In God, whose word I praise, in God I have put my trust; I shall not be afraid." I placed my fears at His feet, choosing to trust Him again.

My then eight-month-old grandson, unable to walk by himself, always raised his hands to be held and carried when he couldn't get somewhere on his own. I loved this about him and couldn't help but think, isn't this how we should be with God, reaching up to Him for help knowing we cannot make it on our own? Those days I often found myself simply praying, "Help!"—the shortest prayer I know, but one of me simply raising my hands and asking the Lord to carry me through.

A Letter from My Husband

Monday morning, two days before my scheduled mastectomy, I woke to find this letter from my husband waiting for me at the breakfast table:

Dearest Camilla,

I will not ask you to be unafraid. Whether marine, teacher, sailor, nurse, or wife and mother, there will be a time to fear. Yet, it is how we face fear that distinguishes the courageous from the cowardly.

"A coward dies a thousand times before his death, but the valiant only once. The military man, facing chaos and death, despite fear, does his duty. Duty is ours, the consequences are God's."
– Thomas J. (Stonewall) Jackson

The beloved wife and mother, facing the loss of a part of her femininity, despite fear, undergoes breast surgery. She does what is right and what has been determined to be medically necessary, not only for her sake but for those she loves. Even though she walks through the valley of the shadow of death, she fears no evil for God is with her. Like Job, she says, "though He slay me, yet shall I trust Him."

"There is, in addition to a courage with which men die, a courage by which men must live."
– John F. Kennedy

"You gain strength, courage, and confidence by every experience in which you really stop to look fear in the face. You must do the thing you think you cannot do." –Eleanor Roosevelt

Camilla, you can face this surgery only through Christ, who gives you strength. Know, my dear, that you are loved! After this surgery, there will be less of you to love, but you will not be loved any less.

You are loved by many friends, you are loved by family, you are loved by me, and, most importantly, you are loved with an everlasting love—by the almighty God Who is love!

I pray that the peace of God which transcends all understanding will guard your heart and mind in Christ Jesus. Cam, when you are weak, He is strong!

Therefore, Camy, be strong and courageous! For the God of all hope and comfort has said, I will never leave you or forsake you.

God is with you always!

Your loving husband, who will be with you too,

– Bob

His encouragement gave me the courage to face this surgery. I could feel his prayers as well as the prayers of countless other family members and friends because, beyond all understanding, as the days led up to my surgery I felt all of my fears melt away.

Someone Is Praying for You

Through my cancer journey, countless people told me they were praying for me. Often people would say they wished they could do more than pray. What could be more than earnestly storming Heaven's gates to the all-knowing Almighty God on my behalf?! I heard a preacher say the reason most prayers aren't answered is that they aren't prayed. It is easy to say we're going to pray for someone, but then, do we pray? I truly appreciated those sincere prayers that were actually prayed for me and I could honestly feel the help they brought.

After my diagnosis became public, a friend sent me a bracelet with the words "Someone is praying for me" woven on the band. I wore this bracelet often and knew every day that it was true. Though you aren't advised to wear any jewelry during surgery, I kept this bracelet on as I arrived and got ready for the procedure and none of the medical staff said a word about it. The RN who took my vital signs and started my IV worked around

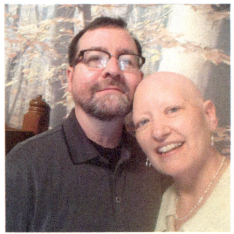
Bob and me with my ugly bald head.

the bracelet and hardly seemed to notice its presence. I know the Lord was with me that day, and I cherished that reminder that many people were praying for me. I was ready for surgery.

As part of the pre-op prep, my plastic surgeon came in and had me stand up naked (all except for my bracelet) in front of him as he sat on a rolling stool. He then took a marker and drew on my chest with the concentration of an artist working on a prized drawing! This was an awkward situation that became commonplace throughout the reconstruction journey.

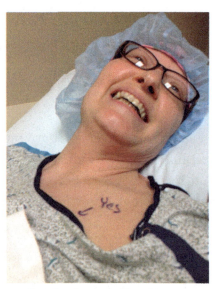
Prepping for my double mastectomy.

While we were discussing reconstruction during an earlier appointment with this surgeon, he grasped my tummy in order to determine how much fat was available and what size my new breasts would be! Bob and I have laughed about this a lot. What was a startling movement to us was "all in a day's work" to my plastic surgeon.

My greatest fear of surgery was still the anesthesia. I was afraid I wouldn't wake up. I also feared I might choke. I have allergies and constantly have drainage in my throat, so what could be done to clear that if I were unconscious? When my anesthesiologist walked into my room, he introduced himself with a name that sounded like "breath." I found this both amusing and comforting, as he was responsible to make sure I kept breathing while sedated. After completing his exam, this compassionate doctor listened to all my fears, reassured me, saying he could clear my throat for me if necessary, and even prayed with us! His prayer brought me the final bit of comfort I needed to face my greatest fear. I was privileged to have him in charge of my breathing for my first and last breast surgeries.

When I woke up I would no longer have my power port or either of my breasts.

Feeling Drained

After my cancer treatment started, one of the first things Bob would say when he got home from work was, "How do you feel today?" I had often replied with words like:

- Zapped
- Achy
- Icky
- Yucky
- Tired

- Miserable
- So, so
- Okay
- Not so bad
- Crummy

- Pre-nauseous
- Nauseous
- Hollow
- Lost
- Weak

The day after surgery I chose to feel "thankful to be alive." Even now when we drive by the hospital where I had my bilateral mastectomy, my first thought is, "That's where I lost my breasts." Before the thought is complete, though, I change it to, "That's where my life was spared." We can choose to be grumpy or grateful.

After the mastectomy my range of motion was limited, and my arms a little sore. I was sent home after one night's stay with Valium (diazepam) and Oxycontin (oxycodone), which alleviated my pain with minimal unwanted side effects.

What was most uncomfortable, though, were the Jackson-Pratt (JP) drains. I had two attached to each side of my chest. These were long tubes which dangled out of my body from the surgical sites; suction bulbs were attached at the end of each tube. They were inserted to collect fluid from around the surgery area. The drains were secured with a few sutures, which if pulled, would really sting. I found wearing a zip up hoodie was helpful as I could store the drains within the front pockets. Also, with the limited range of motion in my arms, zip or button up tops were easiest to put on. While showering, I would wrap the JP drains around my neck to keep them from pulling.

Once we arrived home from the hospital, Bob's job was to strip and empty the drains. The fluid in each drain, as well as its color and density, had to be measured and recorded.

The medical team told me my job was to rest. It was difficult to feel rested while I had two long tubes dangling out either side of my chest. I knew I still needed God's help even in my resting. I found comfort in Matthew 11:28-29, "Come to Me, all who are weary and heavy-laden, and I will give you rest. Take My yoke upon you and learn from Me, for I am gentle and humble in heart, and you will find rest for your souls."

My discharge orders included a few exercises for me in order to gain back my strength and mobility. My favorite and most helpful one was what I termed the "I Dream of Jeannie" pose—stretching my arms over my head and clasping my hands together (like pretending to be a church steeple). It seemed to combine all the exercises into one and the stretch felt good.

Since my breasts were small, a mere 34A, some might say a mastectomy for me should have been less of a big deal, as if I had less to lose. But these were *my* breasts, and the loss I felt was big.

The cancer was only in my right breast, but we decided to remove both breasts to decrease the odds of getting breast cancer all over again! Another reason to do a bilateral mastectomy was, as one doctor put it, so my "reconstruction would look more symmetrical."

I had two surgeons operate on me during my mastectomy. My breast surgeon removed my breasts, cancerous skin, and lymph nodes. She was responsible to prepare the removed body parts for testing. She also removed the power port.

Then my plastic surgeon took over, inserting tissue expanders where my breasts used to be. Tissues expanders are empty breast implants, used to temporarily hold the place for permanent reconstruction. The expanders were placed on top of my pectoral muscles and acellular dermal matrix was used to keep them in place. These expanders, even before being inflated, were close to my original breasts' size, so with bandages on I looked "normal."

I had heard stories that mastectomy patients' worst moment was seeing themselves naked in a mirror for the first time post-surgery. My experience with this, however, wasn't so bad, maybe because, since being warned about this event, I was more mentally prepared for it. My first peek couldn't happen for about a week, though, as the final bandages didn't come off until the first post-op appointment.

We returned to my plastic surgeon's office five days after surgery for my post-op appointment, and I was excited to have one set of those pesky surgical drains removed. First the surgeon clipped the stitches holding the tube in place. Then he gently tugged and pulled out the tube. I had a queasy sensation as the tube traveled a surprisingly long distance through my body. Into the waste basket it went as the nurse was standing close to my side to receive it. They repeated the process on the second one, with the added shock of us all getting sprayed as fluid unexpectantly spewed out with the tube on its way to the trash!

My chest bandage was also removed then, and I was given a stretchy pink flowered breast binder (similar to the tube tops we wore in the 1970s) to wear. This gave some support for the expanders and added a little pressure for complete healing of the breast incisions.

After that post-op appointment, the moment had finally come for me to study myself naked. Upon my first viewing, I mourned the loss of my nipples, had a few tears, then thanked God I was alive and had the opportunity of reconstruction. My incisions were smooth horizontal straight lines across each breast, I was impressed at the thin, flat scar. These incisions were mostly healed and no longer hurt. My breast mounds looked awkward to me at first without nipples, but knowing I would have some form of nipples someday after reconstruction helped me adjust to this new me.

The drainage tube sites were still painful, but I was able to reduce my pain meds and do a little more activity each day, like needle work, walking around the house, light housework, and cooking.

Though my breasts were completely gone, the strangest side effect I experienced, and may continue to experience for as long as I live, is a phantom itch in my "breasts" that I can't scratch. I have heard of people who've had a foot amputated and would continue to feel pain in that missing foot. Now I found myself experiencing the same thing—my mind reaching out for a part of my body that was no longer there.

By this time, it had been about four months since I lost my hair. I noticed little tiny eyelashes starting to grow, a few eyebrow hairs appearing, and peach fuzz all over my head!

Gradually, I started feeling better and participating more in life. It's interesting how we continue to adjust to our new normals. Hinderances become our current situation as we learn how to deal with them. I would have days where I thought I was going backwards instead of forwards in recovery, but I found that was common with any surgery.

The last set of drains came out one week after the first. I continued to meet weekly with my plastic surgeon to check my incisions. Soon they had sufficiently healed to take on pressure. My plastic surgeon began adding air, a little at a time, into my expanders. This process continued at appointments one to two weeks apart. The doctor expanded as long as there was no infection or wounds.

Filling the expanders wasn't a painful procedure at all, as the skin had lost its sensation. The medical staff would use a tool to locate the port part of the expander, then insert a needle in it to add air—like blowing up a balloon.

This slow stretching of my skin was slightly painful, but the result was growing new skin for my reconstruction surgery. The expanders were hard, which felt weird when hugging, but I was appreciative of "breasts" that looked normal under clothes.

The expanding had to stop for radiation. Since my radiation was scheduled to start mid-January, we had plenty of time to get to my desired size. In women who are desiring larger implants, and therefore have larger expanders, sometimes a little deflation is necessary (only for the duration of radiation) if the breast is in the way of a radiation beam.

At three weeks post-op, my breast surgeon released me to most normal activities and gave us the pathology report: "invasive ductal carcinoma, intermediate grade, nuclear grade 3. Metastatic ductal carcinoma to 4 of 11 lymph nodes. The tumor was 4.6x3.2x2.0cm, overall residual viable cancer cellularity (the proportion of cancer) of the tumor bed: 50-60%."

We met with my oncologist, getting more news about my cancer: "ER 100% positive, PR 65% positive, HER2/neu negative, Ki67 1% favorable (PR & Ki67 decreased from chemotherapy.)"

In layman's terms, I had stage 3B invasive cancer in my right breast which had also spread to the skin of the breast and the lymph nodes under my right arm. There wasn't any cancer in my left breast that was also removed during this surgery. Estrogen (ER) and progesterone (PR) positives meant that my cancer would most likely respond to hormonal therapy, which inhibits the production of female hormones and thus the growth of breast cancer cells. Human epidermal growth factor receptor-2 (HER2) negative meant I had slower growing tumors.

Be Strong and Courageous

The decision to surgically remove my breasts took courage. After all, this would be final/permanent, my breasts could not be reattached. I had to trust the decision we made and move forward. This stretched my faith. I needed courage, but how could I get it? The key was to fear God and not my circumstances. This doesn't mean to be afraid of God, but to respect Him. If I really respect Him, I can trust Him to care for me in spite of my circumstances.

The definition of encourage is, "give support, confidence, or hope to someone." As others prayed for me and *encouraged* me, I could proceed. It was like they were giving me the courage I needed.

> "Have I not commanded you? Be strong and courageous! Do not tremble or be dismayed, for the LORD your God is with you wherever you go."
> – Joshua 1:9

CHAPTER 7

Thorny Ways Lead to a Joyful End

Be Still

" The machine will sound like an airplane taking off," my radiation therapist said. She was referring to the CT scan that was taking images during my radiation treatment planning session. My radiation oncologist, along with a radiation physicist, determined the exact treatment area for my radiation. My doctor then made four dot tattoos with a very small needle and drop of ink. These are permanent tattoos, marking the area of the radiation field. This allowed precise and consistent placement of the radiation beam. I never thought I would be getting tattoos—another first!

Tattoos given, pictures taken, equipment shown, and side effects explained; all systems were go for my six weeks of radiation. My sessions were Monday through Friday at 11:00 AM—as if I wasn't going to the doctor enough already!

Coming in for a landing, I found myself at church the following Sunday taking in the soothing melody of "Be Still My Soul" playing softly in the background as we prepared to worship. In light of the radiation I would face in the coming six weeks, the song seemed very fitting:

Be still, my soul: the Lord is on thy side.

> [Be still. That's what the technician told me to do as she positioned me on the table. The beams had to align just right to prevent the radiation from damaging healthy parts of the body. As we waited for the first radiation session to begin, Meridith and I quoted the verse that had been on our minds through this whole cancer journey: "'Do not fear, for I am with you; do not anxiously look about you, for I am your God. I will strengthen you, surely I will help you, surely I will uphold you with My righteous right hand'" (Isaiah 41:10). These words eased the fear that gripped my heart.]

Bear patiently the cross of grief or pain.

> [The tech explained the walls around the radiation room were a five-foot thick concoction of lead and concrete. The techs would line me up correctly according to my tattoos, double check my position, then leave the room. It was an eerie feeling being left in this huge room under a very large radiation machine. I could hear the heavy door latch shut. I was all alone. I felt isolated, separated from the rest of the world. In that moment my mind went to Jesus being separated from God as He hung on the cross. Then I remembered that Jesus was *truly* alone at that time, as God had to forsake Him as they completed the sacrifice of His blood removing our sins. Even though I *felt* all alone, I wasn't alone, as God was with me. That is what made this next treatment procedure bearable.]

Leave to thy God to order and provide;

> [Though radiation can cause harmful effects to the skin and potentially other parts of the body, I had to trust that God would guide my radiation oncologist, physicist, and techs as they planned and performed the treatments. I needed to believe He would guide afterwards regardless of the outcome.]

In every change, He faithful will remain.
>[*Radiation was the new leg of this cancer marathon, bringing with it scary unknowns, but God has promised to never leave or forsake us.*]

Be still, my soul: thy best, thy heavenly Friend
Through thorny ways leads to a joyful end.
>[*Although the daily trips seemed unending, they led to eradication of cancer cells.*]

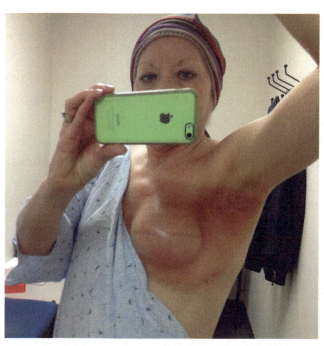

Still a week to go with daily radiations. The thin straight-line scar is a result of the mastectomy and expander insertions.

Radiation had fewer side effects than chemotherapy. I definitely got fatigued, a tiredness that sleep couldn't alleviate. My radiated site, right breast area and underarm, got angry red and irritated. At the end of my six weeks of radiation my skin looked like it was severely sunburned. It was uncomfortable but not extreme. CeraVe lotion was soothing; my radiation oncologist also prescribed Biafine and RadiaGel topical ointments. The hair in my underarm area never did grow back, and it often peels like a sunburn.

My thirty radiation treatments had left me feeling zapped, but I was grateful to have another piece of my cancer treatment done.

Peace

It was time for a checkup with my oncologist. He prescribed Nolvadex (tamoxifen), a selective estrogen receptor modulator. This hormonal or endocrine therapy was the second part of my systemic (whole body) therapy, chemotherapy being the first. Tamoxifen is one of the breast cancer drugs I would need to take for ten years. Five years was the recommended time when I was diagnosed with breast cancer, but new research revealed ten years as opposed to five is the best scenario. I started taking tamoxifen after a body rest from radiation.

Tamoxifen caused annoying hot flashes that would come on suddenly and soak my clothes. Interesting positive side effects, though: tamoxifen can lower cholesterol and increase bone density.

After one year of no menstrual periods, thus confirming my arrival at menopause, my oncologist planned to switch me to an aromatase inhibitor. According to research, the aromatase inhibitors are more effective at fighting my type of cancer but not safe for women who could become pregnant.

A few weeks leading up to this appointment I had a foggy, fuzzy brain. I was having trouble getting my mind to focus—similarly to my grocery list struggles. I wasn't my sharp self. I would forget peoples' names, common words while conversing, and what I was saying mid-sentence. I would suddenly see tasks not completed that I had completely forgotten to finish. I didn't need to ask Bob about this as he had noticed my deficiencies as well. After discussing with my oncologist, he ordered a brain CT scan. This was a reasonable caution "in the off-chance cancer has moved there and to put our minds at ease."

As I waited for the results of the brain CT, I found comfort in Isaiah 26:3: "The steadfast of mind You will keep in perfect peace, because he trusts in You." I knew that whatever the outcome, God would see me through; He had proven that on this journey over and over already.

Soon I got the CT scan results:
1. "No definite evidence of intracranial metastatic disease."

(There was no sign that the breast cancer had spread to my brain.)

2. "Small likely extra-axial enhancing lesion along the anterior aspect of the right sphenoid wing which is slightly hyperdense on the pre-contrast images. This most likely represents a small partially calcified meningioma."

(There was, however, a benign growth in my brain that needed to be watched.)

The plan was to rescan or do an MRI in three months. An MRI is more accurate in detecting brain cancer, but uses a strong magnetic field. Therefore, I couldn't have an MRI as long as the metal expanders were in my chest.

I have been asked if I was anxious about the possibility of brain cancer. My brother often says, "It is what it is." Somehow, I found comfort in that statement. God had given me peace even in the waiting.

Hair I Am

By the end of February 2016, my eyebrows and eyelashes had grown back to their pre-chemo state.

When I was first facing the thought of losing all of my hair, a friend encouraged me by saying, "God knows how many hairs to put back because they are all numbered; what an awesome detail!" She was right. We read this in Mathew 10:30.

Now, my hair, which had come in all gray, had grown enough to get a haircut and style.

I had never had hair this short! I walked in the salon with a hat on. I left sporting my new haircut, going out in public for the first time in several months with an uncovered head. After having long hair for so many years, I really did feel conspicuous and masculine. The very last time that I had short hair was when I was seventeen. I'd had it cut, without Mom's permission, before my month-long trip to Europe. I was told it would be easier to care for that way. Boy, was that bad advice for me! It couldn't grow out fast enough! I found short hair more laborious as drying and styling every morning was a must. With long hair, I could wash it the night before, letting it air dry overnight. When there wasn't time to use hot rollers or a curling iron, a ponytail or bun was a quick style. Also, bedhead wasn't an issue with long hair, so daily washing wasn't necessary.

I had blonde hair as a child, and for the past several years I'd had blonde highlights added to my hair. And now here I was, all of a sudden, with gray hair!! Gray hair was a little scary, but my stylist said, "Gray hair is now in." She advised me not to color my hair. I eventually got used to my hair being gray and even started to like it.

The night of that first short gray haircut, Bob and I went out to dinner to celebrate being done with radiation. I had made the reservation under my husband's name. Upon checking in, the host said, "You don't look like a Robert!" He had no idea how applicable and timely that comment was and how happy it made me.

I have always been most comfortable and felt most natural with long hair, but there I was with a very short hairstyle! Everyone told me how cute it was, and I truly appreciated and needed their encouragement. However, I just didn't feel like me in short hair. I'd go to my stylist every four to six weeks, and she'd work her magic, cutting, experimenting, and styling as it slowly grew to varying lengths. Finally, on May 9, 2018, I was able to make a pony tail again—a happy dance day for me!

When I tell people about losing my hair, I often say, "It came back short and gray." Duh! Of course, it came in short!

Loose Ends

One very normal morning after showering I chose from my closet an ordinary shirt that I hadn't worn in a long time. Nothing in particular was on my mind. After pulling it over my head and putting my arms through, I discovered one of my old long hairs in the right sleeve! I was so excited I removed it to measured it—twenty-two inches! Obviously, it was a shirt I hadn't worn since before chemotherapy took my long hair! What used to be a regular itchy annoyance, became a sweet reflection of years gone by. My stylist and I figured out that my hair grows 1/4 inch per month, so it would take over seven years to get that long again!

It was then that I realized that I was content with my post-cancer hair. In fact, I often received compliments on the gray color—and it was totally God given. When my hair had grown to just below my neck, I really liked it and was contented with this length. I also discovered through our hairstyle experimentation that my face looked good with bangs. I hadn't had bangs since childhood.

My new favorite length took about three years to grow. I finally liked the way my hair looked again. I liked the way my hair felt on me. I had found a favorable hairstyle again. It made me feel cheery, jovial. Funny how our hair can make us happy! But, really, around this time I had realized I was more content overall. God's refining was doing its work; the process of going through breast cancer was changing me. I even had people tell me I seemed happier. I was coming to the end, and it was true, as the old hymn says, "through thorny ways leads to a joyful end."

CHAPTER 8

Reconstruction

Trans-Fat

Fat generally gets a bad rap as being unhealthy. There are endless weight loss articles, TV shows, apps. People sometimes spend months or even years, trying to burn belly fat. After breast reconstruction surgery, my belly fat disappeared, not in years or months, but in hours—nine, to be exact. I don't say this to brag but to introduce yet another rapid transformation in my body during this cancer journey. Ironically, post-surgery setbacks led to the removal of every milligram of fat from my diet. Additional setbacks would come, and regular life annoyances would stack on top of these. But still, God remained faithful, patiently reconstructing me spiritually, even as my body was being reconstructed physically.

As a prosthesis is fitted after a leg amputation, the goal of breast reconstruction is to restore what was lost due to cancer treatment.

> *The goal of breast reconstruction is to restore what was lost due to cancer treatment.*

DIEP flap reconstruction is a major surgery with risks. In fact, those first few nights after surgery are spent in the intensive care unit (ICU). The recovery time is eight weeks. My plastic surgeon joked that I would hate him immediately, but love him later.

First, the surgeon would remove my expanders. He would then use a tedious technique to separate the skin, fat, and blood vessels in my abdomen and shape them into my new "breasts." Using microsurgery, the doctor would reconnect the new breasts to the blood supply in the chest. My belly button would have to be moved; otherwise, it would end up in a weird place. My abdomen would then be sewn up, stretching the skin to make up for the few inches removed with the fat. This is a lot to do to my body just so I could have breasts again!

After many appointments with my plastic surgeon explaining the DIEP flap reconstruction, discussions with others who had had the same procedure, internet research, and talking it over with family, I decided to go through with it. The major factor convincing me was that my breasts would be made from my own body tissue and not foreign objects; I wouldn't have the risks associated with breast implants.

But, as the time drew nearer, I started to get more and more nervous. Going under anesthesia for several hours, putting my body through a grueling surgery, and thinking of the necessary recovery time afterwards all left me feeling uneasy.

Graciously, God provided interruptions and events leading up to the date that kept me sufficiently busy, leaving little time to dwell on and worry about what lay ahead. First, a college roommate I hadn't seen in over thirty years was passing through my city, and we were able to catch up over breakfast. This is the Christian friend I was living with when I got saved. Back then she spent countless hours answering my many questions and discipling me. As a result, she has always been near and dear to my heart. Another happy interruption was our military son being able to make it home for a short visit. Our daughter was also here, and our oldest son and family live locally, so all the Cranks were together for a couple of days. Many other friends and family "randomly" called me to join them for events or have a meal with them—all of which took my mind off the upcoming surgery.

Tuesday April 26, 2016, the morning of my DIEP flap surgery arrived, and I was grateful to have Bob and Meridith by my side once again. All the prep happened, including standing naked in front of the plastic surgeon so he could draw on me again!

The surgery began around 8:45 AM. About every two hours, a nurse would update Bob and Meridith on the surgeon's progress. The fat separation took the whole morning and into the afternoon. Meridith later told me that when they received their last update that the fat had been transferred to the upper chest and the surgeon was reconnecting all the blood vessels, they breathed a huge sigh of relief—knowing the worst part was over.

Finally, around 5:45 PM, they were told that my surgery was completed. I remember waking up from surgery as I was being wheeled to the ICU. I could see Bob and Meridith out of the corner of my eye. I wanted to greet them, but the nurse told them to wait a few minutes while they got me settled. Seeing their faces was a welcome sight. I appreciated that they were willing to wait at the hospital as I was operated on for so many hours. Having them there when I was wheeled into surgery and knowing they would be there when I awoke, gave me great comfort. It was a short day for me but a long day for them!

I was so sleepy, in pain, and basically out of it, but once Bob and Meridith were allowed in my room, we visited a bit. They told me my plastic surgeon said, "I think Camy will be pleased with the results." I kept asking them to tell me again as I was wanting reassurance that everything turned out well.

After a while Bob left for home, but Meridith decided to spend the night with me. "I thought I should probably return home with Dad to get a more restful sleep," she said, "but the nurse in me couldn't be pulled away from that ICU room. I wanted to watch the trend in Mom's vital signs and see firsthand that she was still breathing."

The first twelve to forty-eight hours would reveal whether the skin grafts and reconnected vessels withstood the transfer. It was a busy night with the hourly monitoring of the grafts, listening to the blood vessels in my breasts with a doppler similar to what is used to hear a baby's heartbeat in the womb. I also had vital sign checks every fifteen to thirty minutes. They say you don't go to the hospital to get sleep and that certainly held true this first night! Anytime I dozed off, an alarm jerked me awake. I was hooked up to oxygen, and the alarm signaled I wasn't getting enough. Meridith would then remind me to take some deep breaths through my nose to silence the alarm.

Around 10 PM, my blood pressure began to drop, most likely due to the epidural that was helping to relieve my pain. Eventually, the anesthesiologist decided to discontinue the epidural completely, hoping my blood pressure would rise again.

Due to the trauma to the abdomen during the surgery, the physician ordered strict bedrest for the first twenty-four hours. Flat on my back, head elevated to thirty degrees (no more, no less), and no turning from side to side whatsoever.

I had the whole painful drain thing going again, only more this time as they were not only coming out the side of each new breast, but also each side of my abdomen as well. I remember a thunderstorm throughout the night and thinking it would be nice to get up and look out the window, but I could barely move, let alone get out of bed!

By 10 AM, my blood pressure finally evened out to a more normal level, easing Meridith's concern. But day two was more difficult for other reasons. I couldn't wait to get out of bed, but as soon as the nurse sat me up on the side of the bed, I asked to lie back down! The nausea and pain were intense. I've heard that abdominal surgery is one of the worst. I can attest that it sure hurts! Since they took out several inches of my stomach skin, my abdomen was so tight that once I did stand up I was completely hunched over! On top of that I had chest congestion, and I couldn't get the mucus coughed up due to the pain. I was a definite baby when it came to coughing. It hurt so badly in my belly I felt like I was going to split open.

Eventually we adjusted the timing of my nausea medications so that their effectiveness coincided to when the nurses would sit me on the side of the bed. After success with that, I was able to sit in a chair beside the bed. Then I got my urine catheter removed and was able to walk to the bathroom, then walk across the room to sit in a chair. By day four I was up walking the halls, anticipating going home.

Can't Breathe

Before getting released, however, I had a little setback. Saturday my doctor ordered a chest CT scan, as I still had congestion and still needed oxygen. Meridith was granted permission to accompany me to the test but then told to stand outside the procedure room. As soon as the tech began lowering my body on the CT scan bed, I felt like I was suffocating and frantically whispered, "I can't breathe!" Meridith was immediately by my side, raising me up and helping me catch my breath. I was terrified, and I felt as though I was drowning. I have never been afraid of cancer, but have always been afraid of drowning. After being reconnected to oxygen and improvising with pillows to get me into a semi-reclined position, the techs were able to complete the scan. The entire five minutes I kept repeating, "God, please help me breathe!"

In his familiar dedication, my plastic surgeon wasted no time relaying the results. There weren't any blood clots in my lungs; however, fluid was surrounding them, and I had atelectasis (the bases of the lungs hadn't fully expanded since surgery.) Both of these conditions weren't life-threatening, but they made it difficult to breathe. He prescribed Lasix (furosemide) to help get the fluid off.

When Meridith left the hospital to go to church Sunday, I was determined to stop being a baby and cough up the gunk in my lungs. The nurse said to push my pain pump for a MorphaBond (morphine) dose, then hug a pillow and cough. My first attempts were wimpy. I could barely muster an "ahem." No way was it deep enough to loosen the mucus. After several attempts, I finally had some productive coughs.

Home Sweet Home

I was in the hospital for five nights. When I came home, Meridith and Bob made a bed for me on the couch. There I could wedge myself between the back and bottom cushions, causing less jiggles or jerks on my sensitive incisions and drain exits. I wore a compression garment around my abdomen and an adjustable surgical support bra. Upon discharge my surgeon prescribed a pill form of morphine, oxycodone, and Valium for pain management. I had no idea they would send me home with such potent drugs. I had never been a fan of medications. These powerful ones were especially scary to me, so I wanted to get my body clear of them as soon as possible.

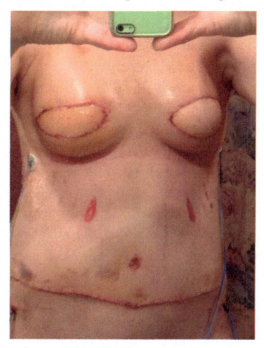
One week after DIEP Flap reconstruction surgery.

You Are an Enigma

After I had been home for a few days, Meridith and I noticed that one breast drain started putting out a strawberry-colored milky substance at an increased rate. One day it produced almost one quart of drainage, ten times the normal amount! Meridith called the doctor's office to report this and was told this sometimes happens. Apparently, the medical person Meridith spoke with didn't fully understand what she was trying to explain because the next day when we went in for my post-op appointment my doctor was aghast with the amount of output we had recorded. He stepped back, stared at me lost in thought, and said, "I think you have a lymph leak."

Looking back, I remember the last nurse I had in the hospital asked her charge nurse why my drainage on that breast had turned milky. Her boss seemed to think that it wasn't too out-of-the-ordinary. It could have been that the charge nurse had simply never seen this before. "You are an enigma!" my doctor said. Later, he also called me a "conundrum." This suspected lymph leak left my plastic surgeon feeling perplexed, as this had never happened before with any of his hundreds of DIEP flap surgeries. He promptly ordered labs, a chest CT scan, and testing of the fluid from the drain. If the breast kept swelling, he said I was to return immediately. This condition could lead to the loss of one of my new "breasts."

Meridith had to catch a flight back to Minnesota the afternoon of my post-op appointment. She and I had some fun plans for our last day together, following what was supposed to be a routine appointment, but our fun never happened. We hurried from my doctor's office to the lab for blood work, then drove to another location for a CT Scan. As we were headed to lunch, my plastic surgeon called to report that both tests confirmed "lymph leak." He wanted me back to his office ASAP, so he could extract the fluid. We had to get Meridith quickly home so she could pack. After saying quick goodbyes, Bob and I returned to the doctor's office, while a devoted neighbor drove Meridith to the airport.

Once we arrived back at the doctor's office, my plastic surgeon manipulated my breast in such a way to empty the extra fluid. He then stuffed rolled-up gauze into the side of my bra to create pressure on the cavity, hoping to prevent it from filling up again. He prescribed Vibramycin (doxycycline), an antibiotic as well as a Lidocaine Patch for the sore drain site. The next morning, we were alarmed to find my breast swollen yet again, so Bob and I immediately headed back to the plastic surgeon's office.

Since the beginning of my cancer diagnosis, I would write personally applicable scriptures friends had sent or that I had found during my Bible study times on index cards. I would carry these verses with me to read during treatments, appointments, and before surgeries. I decided to read my cards aloud to comfort us as we drove to this appointment. Isaiah 58:8-

9a randomly came up first: "Then your light will break out like the dawn, and your recovery will speedily spring forth; and your righteousness will go before you; the glory of the LORD will be your rear guard. Then you will call, and the LORD will answer; you will cry, and He will say, 'Here I am.'" Just being reminded that God was hearing our prayers and that His glory would be our rear guard, protection from unsuspected attack from the encroaching enemy, gave such great comfort to us.

At this visit, after my plastic surgeon extracted the fluid, he stuck tape around my breast for additional pressure. Next, he replaced the original rolled up gauze, adding more for extra measure. Lastly, my surgeon put me on a fat-free diet and instructed us on what to look and feel for in case there was another flair up. I felt like a silly school girl walking out of his office with a stuffed bra!

As we began our search for what I could eat, we were surprised to find fat in almost everything in the American diet! All meat has some fat, so I mostly drank my protein. My favorite was skim milk with Carnation Breakfast Essentials Powder mixed in. One friend found a loaf of bread without fat (of course, I had to eat it without butter—one of my favorite condiments). All fruits and vegetables were okay as long as they remained in their natural state. Not many snacks were available except plain pretzels. Another friend loaned me an air popcorn popper, but then we realized that popcorn has fat, even without cooking it in oil or adding the butter! With a diet like this, as you can imagine, I lost weight almost immediately!

After a few days on the no-fat diet, and extra pressure applied to my breast with the tape and gauze, my breast didn't have any more swelling episodes. It looked like the danger of losing my new breast had passed. When I realized that, I broke out in thanks to the Lord right along with the Psalmist: "Then they cried out to the LORD in their trouble; He saved them out of their distresses. He sent His word and healed them, and delivered them from their destructions. Let them give thanks to the LORD for His lovingkindness, and for His wonders to the sons of men! Let them also offer sacrifices of thanksgiving, and tell of His works with joyful singing" (Psalm 107:19-22). I knew it was the Lord who ultimately brought about my healing, and all I wanted to do in response was tell of His works with joy. *Hallelujah! Thank You, Jesus! How many breasts can one woman lose anyway?*

The doctor removed the tape, now the only treatment left for my lymph leak was the gauze stuffed bra and another two weeks on the no-fat diet! When that two-week period was up, I met with my plastic surgeon again. He was fairly confident the lymph leak was healed. He was pleased to note that all my incisions looked good. He gave me permission to sleep on my side, and I only had to wear the abdominal brace when I felt I needed the support. I no longer needed to stuff my bra! Ah, sleeping on my side (my favorite sleeping position) never felt so good!

My biggest question to the surgeon, though, was, "How do we know *for sure* the lymph leak is healed?" He said you only know it's gone if your body stops producing the extra chyle (lymph). He suggested I gradually begin adding fat to my diet. "No deep-dish pizza," he said. So, I began with lean meats and enjoyed some butter on my toast. We had to be vigilant in watching for a recurrence of the lymph liquid, which would pool in the left breast. Adding some fat back into my diet would allow us to look for that.

Meanwhile, my plastic surgeon did some research on the topic and couldn't find anything written about this complication following the DIEP flap surgery, so he began documenting my case, wrote an article about my lymph leak, and got it published in February 2019. I guess I truly *am* a medical conundrum!

While the worst seemed to be behind me, I still had to keep inching toward the finish line. I continued to wear the support bra for two more weeks, and, though mostly healed, I was still not allowed to lift anything over ten pounds or do any strenuous activity. The hardest part of this was not being able to lift my grandson.

Now it was time for blood work and a follow-up with my oncologist. He said my labs looked good, considering everything I had been through. He agreed with the surgeon on the lymph leak: "Don't get a greasy hamburger and wash it down with a milkshake!"

As each week progressed, I continued to gain back strength and add a few daily chores into my life. Even though I don't particularly enjoy changing the bed sheets or vacuuming, it felt great to do my usual chores. When my morphine prescription ended, I adjusted pretty well to just oxycodone and Valium. I made myself a weaning schedule—counting the number of pills I had left and stretching the time out between taking each one—so I would be off all my prescription pain medications six weeks after my surgery.

> *I made myself a weaning schedule—counting the number of pills I had left and stretching the time out between taking each one—so I would be off all my prescription pain medications six weeks after surgery.*

Final Touches

After I healed from DIEP flap surgery, my plastic surgeon and I discussed how my right breast was smaller than the left due to thicker and less pliable skin caused from the radiation on that side of my chest. He explained more about the Liposuction Fat Transfer procedure. Liposuction is performed on a part of the body that has extra fat; the extracted fat is reconditioned, then it is inserted by syringe needles to the areas that need more fullness.

We decided to liposuction fat from my stomach and flanks. The conditioned fat was added to the smaller right breast. Fat was also inserted in the concave where my port had been and in the indentation where a drain from my right breast had exited my body. Additionally, my surgeon flattened the "dog ears" at each end of my abdominal scar. All of this was outpatient surgery and didn't take long. I was sent home with oxycodone and doxycycline. The donor area was painful, but the areas that received the new fat didn't hurt at all. I was wrapped in a compression garment that I wore for six weeks and had a two-week no-lifting ban. This surgery was in December of 2016.

I had a second Liposuction Fat Transfer six months later. This time they took the fat from my inner thighs. The leg liposuction was much more painful than the abdominal one. I awoke with a compression garment from just under my breasts to just under my knees. The incisions from where the cannula (tube) was inserted were covered with absorption pads and continued to ooze for a couple of days. I had a lot of extra swelling after this surgery and took longer to heal. My legs hurt with common movements, like climbing into bed, kneeling, squatting, or sitting with my legs crossed.

My third and last Liposuction Fat Transfer was six months after the second one in December of 2017, as my right breast was *still* smaller than the left even after the second transfer had healed. This time, fat was taken from my stomach area again.

The whole body swelling from all three liposuctions was very slow to dissipate; I was swollen for over a year after my last surgery. My plastic surgeon added a new description to my growing list of titles: "You continue to be an anatomical anomaly!"

Apparently the excessive swelling I had with my Liposuction Fat Transfer surgeries was unique. The doctor said his patients typically have more bruising and less swelling; mine was the opposite. He drained some extra fluid from the right breast, then instructed me to elevate my legs at night and daytime when possible. I had to continue wearing the compression garments, adding compression socks to my lovely wardrobe. He also gave me another antibiotic prescription, refilled the pain pills, and said to include Advil (ibuprofen) in my arsenal of meds. All of this warranted extra tests with my Lymphedema nurse and extra checkups with my plastic surgeon, but the swelling finally abated. I was excited that my wedding ring finally fit again!

Ever since these procedures, it has been hard to find a bra that fits well; my lymphedema nurse said that many of her breast cancer patients complain about this dilemma. According to a bra specialist, I am now a size 34B. I have found though, that 34C fits me better. In exercise bras, I have had to buy a size large and even extra-large to get a comfortable fit!

My plastic surgeon cautioned me from the start that reconstruction could be a long, drawn-out process. He urged me to be patient and particular, making sure I was satisfied before I finally told him I was done. I appreciate his advice, and I applaud insurance companies for paying for breast reconstruction. After all, if a person loses an arm to cancer, insurance covers a replacement.

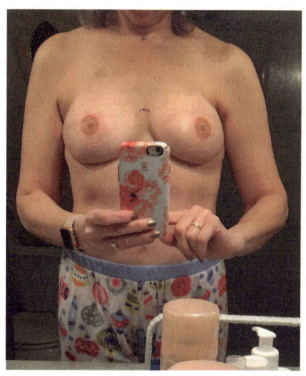

3-D tattooing of nipple and areola. The final step of reconstruction.

I was glad I went through with all three liposuction fat transfers, as my breasts were finally symmetrical. I am very pleased at how my breasts turned out. It felt great having the look and feel of real breasts again. Although difficult to lose my true breasts, it was a clean feeling, knowing my cancerous breast was gone. Without realizing it, I had begun referring to these breast mounds as my breasts. The final touch would be "nipples." Then they would look as real without clothes on as they did with clothes on.

That's Tat

When discussing the nipple options, my surgeon said the most popular now is 3-D nipple/areola tattooing only. This skips the step of actually cutting, molding, and stitching an erect nipple on each breast. He said the molded nipple procedure can fail after a few years and also makes wearing a padded bra essential as the nipples are always erect. In the 3-D tattooing-only method, the nipple and areola are tattooed in such a way that it looks like you have protruding nipples, when in actuality they are flat. A perk of this method is that you can go braless without looking immodest. Taking the advice of my plastic surgeon, the 3-D tattooing-only method is the one I chose.

Bob and I met for a one-hour consultation in my plastic surgeon's office where the tech explained the procedure, helped us pick the pigment that matched my skin, and suggested size then placement of the nipple and areola. She then started the actual tattooing process, which took another hour. There wasn't much pain, as not all, but most feeling was gone from my breasts.

Tattooing could also be done outside the hospital setting, but my "medical tattoos" won't interfere with tests and procedures as street tattoos can. The downside of medical tattoos is that they fade and need to be touched-up every two to three years.

The tech told me I needed to brag to my kids about having tattoos! We also were commenting about the by-gone "bad" stigma of tattoos and the coolness of their use in the medical field. The connotation has changed. We used to think people with tattoos were rebellious or immoral. I've come to realize that we are all broken and we are all terminal—none of us are getting out of here alive—unless we're talking about the rapture (even so, come LORD Jesus!).

It just so happened that I was having this final procedure done on Easter weekend. As we reflected on the finished work of Jesus' death and resurrection, I kept hearing the phrase, "It is finished!" Yes, I was thrilled and relieved that my breast reconstruction was finished! Even more than that, though, my atonement for sin was taken care of once and for all the moment Jesus cried out "It is finished" from the cross. My sin has been erased, and I can rely on God's help now and forevermore. Hallelujah what a Savior! IT IS FINISHED!!

Semper Gumby

"Semper Fidelis" is the United States Marine Corps motto; it means "always faithful." When Kevin attended the United States Naval Academy, our family motto became "Semper Gumby" (remember that flexible green guy with his orange horse, Pokey?). "Semper Gumby," meaning "always flexible" because circumstances or plans could, and did, change often. We had to remain adaptable and go with the flow.

Flexibility is valuable on any journey as setbacks are common, often progress is slow, and unexpected things happen. That's is life on this earth. As Jesus said in John 16:33b, "In the world you have tribulation, but take courage; I have overcome the world."

Near the beginning of my breast cancer journey, the garbage disposal broke. Yes, really, as if we needed something else to deal with. But you know what? Annoyances still happen even when your life is in the midst of a crisis. A cancer diagnosis doesn't give us a pass on the other problems in life.

We needed a little Semper Gumby here—breast cancer diagnosis, surgery and anesthesia fears, chemotherapy treatment and their side effects, dreaded hair loss, surgical removal of my breasts, radiation, nine-hour reconstruction surgery and recovery. Then we saw God's Semper Fidelis pile up in heaps all around. He not only gave me the strength to get through each of those difficulties, but He turned them into positive experiences. God had heard my cries for help in my distresses and faithfully met each need. I had concrete evidence that God is trustworthy. "You who have shown me many troubles and distresses will revive me again" (Psalm 71:20a).

Half-way through my breast cancer journey my daughter-in-law had this verse framed for me: "Do not fear, for I have redeemed you; I have called you by name; you are Mine! When you pass through the waters, I will be with you; and through the rivers, they will not overflow you. When you walk through the fire, you will not be scorched, nor will the flame burn you" (Isaiah 43:1b-2). While this verse brought me a lot of comfort as I was heading into reconstruction surgery, now, looking back, I can see clearly how true it was. The verse uses the word *when* not, *if*. God didn't *spare* me from the difficulties of life or even the added difficulties that occurred in my breast cancer treatment, but God had been *with* me every step of the way. The Lord is faithful, and I knew I could trust that He is always in control. I belong to Him.

I am reminded of something Elisabeth Elliott said: "While it is perfectly true that some of my worst fears did, in fact, materialize, I see them now as 'an abyss and mass of mercies,' appointed and assigned by a loving and merciful Father who sees the end from the beginning. He asks us to trust him." We can be always flexible because we know God is always faithful.

CHAPTER 9

Treasures Hidden in the Darkness

A Battle for My Husband

Our thirty-first wedding anniversary was December 22, 2015 (what were we thinking, getting married three days before Christmas?). Most years, we went away overnight, which crams one more thing to do into an already busy month. But once we made the plans and left home, everywhere we went was decorated for the holidays. It was so festive and inviting, as if all the hubbub was for us! In 2015, though, we didn't plan a "get away" for two reasons. First, I was tired, having insomnia, and just not feeling too great. Second, ALL our kids planned to be home, so we wanted to enjoy that valuable time together as a family.

Our wedding vows included the common phrase, "for better or for worse, in sickness and in health." At the time of the wedding, we weren't thinking about the worse or sickness scenarios. Through the years, there have been "worse" times, but as we lived through them and worked on forgiving, we found our marriage stronger. When we left the breast surgeon's office with my cancer diagnosis in June, I was sad, scared, and worried. But Bob came leaping out of the building, saying, "I don't care if you lose your hair, I don't care if you lose a breast, I'm not losing you! Did you hear what she said? This is curable! We can fight this!"

Oh, yes! Remember, my husband is a United States Marine! Marines know how to fight; losing is not an option! Marines fight to win! Wow! What an answer! He is committed to the "sickness" part of our vow. He had been living it out those past months. He had been my nurse, laundry man, taxi driver, and Siamese twin at doctor appointments. He had given me unconditional love, strong support to lean on, countless hugs, and reassurance of my purpose in life. He even bought groceries by himself, something he hadn't had to do since we got married. I hit the jackpot in marrying Bob. Just so you know, my husband used to be a Major Crank!— but that only lasted until his next promotion! These past months he had proven to be a rare treasure.

You know what was especially great? Bob and I were not alone in fighting my cancer battle. 2 Chronicles 32:7b-8a says, "...for the One with us is greater than the one with him. With him is only an arm of flesh, but with us is the LORD our God to help us and to fight our battles." Hezekiah, king of Judah, was encouraging his warriors with those words as they were preparing to fight Sennacherib, king of Assyria and the horde that was with him. Because God is our Lord and He commands the angel armies, we also had an army fighting on our behalf. I found that, as scary as it sounds to say, nothing in this life would be too difficult to go through because God would be right there with me.

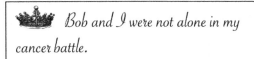
Bob and I were not alone in my cancer battle.

Inside Out

I always thought I was a healthy person, rarely needing to see my doctor except for well-woman checkups. Unbeknownst to me, though, cancer was lurking in my body. On the outside, I looked fine, but inside, I had a major medical issue brewing.

This can be true of our emotional health as well. Outside we can look great, covering up secrets and ghosts from our pasts. In Matthew 23:27 Jesus warns, "Woe to you, scribes and Pharisees, hypocrites! For you are like whitewashed tombs which on the outside appear beautiful, but inside they are full of dead men's bones and all uncleanness."

Nothing is hidden from God's sight. For as Psalm 44:21 says, "Would not God find this out? For He knows the secrets of the heart." The good news is that even though He knows everything about us, He still loves us anyway, as Romans 5:8 states, "But God demonstrates His own love toward us, in that while we were yet sinners, Christ died for us."

My doctors didn't tell me to get well before they would see me. They took me as their patient in my broken, sick state, and came up with a plan to make me better. God takes a sinful, dead person and makes him alive and well. I am very thankful for well-trained physicians, but I am mostly grateful for the Great Physician, Who is able to heal not only my body, but my sinful heart as well.

In the Dark

Now that the expanders were out of my body, my oncologist scheduled an MRI to check on my little brain tumor. The MRI confirmed that the cancer had not gone to my brain. The MRI results also showed my meningioma was "stable"—no change from the previous brain CT scan. While this was great news, I was still feeling down—anxious, sleepy, and depressed most days.

My doctors said it was normal for me to feel this way, considering my year of cancer treatments, followed by Meridith discovering a health crisis of her own. We learned she had a pituitary brain tumor (thankfully not cancerous) and was diagnosed with acromegaly. This required multiple surgeries in her brain and over the course of two years surgeries in both hips as well. On top of that our Navy son was deployed to the middle east. In fact, one doctor said he would be surprised if I *wasn't* having some emotional problems!

My medical team, husband, family, and I tried different avenues in hopes of finding a solution to my feelings. My oncologist prescribed Zoloft (sertraline), an antidepressant, and Ativan (lorazepam), an anti-anxiety medication. I was most anxious about not being able to sleep, so he thought Ativan would relax me and help me sleep. In the meantime, I felt lost. I had spent a year fighting for my life, and now here I was trying to get to know this person who had survived.

The one stable force in my life was, and still is, God. He is my Rock, a Fortress that won't be shaken (Psalm 62:2). I clung to Him. I believed in His faithful presence as I walked that unfamiliar path. I believed in His unlimited power to help me through. I believed in His perfect goodness in all His ways. And I believed in what our twenty-month old grandson sang: "My God is so big, so strong and so mighty! There's nothing my God cannot do!"

This experience showed me that mental illness is not imagined, but real, and heightened my sensitivity to my fellow travelers. We are all broken and struggling with something; not one of us has it all together. Whether I

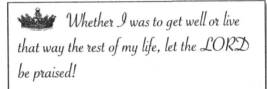
Whether I was to get well or live that way the rest of my life, let the LORD be praised!

was to get well or live that way the rest of my life, let the LORD be praised!

I could have joy in the Lord without feeling joyful. The joy He gave me through my new life in Christ was a fact, not a feeling. Often, I didn't feel it, but that didn't negate its truth. Sometimes I secretly wondered if God had left me; however, I decided to take Him at His word, believing that He was still there with me just as He many times said.

On days I just didn't *feel* like reading the Bible, I read it anyway. The Psalms are an easier place for me to read when I am feeling down and when concentration might be lacking. When I needed to pray, but couldn't, I asked friends to pray *for* me. Listening to hymns or spiritual songs that were more somber was helpful. I chose to just *be*, without expectations of myself or others.

God was with me through the darkness, and He even grew me in it. There was nothing else to cling to but Him, and He proved Himself faithful.

Everything else in life seemed to lose its meaning for me. I was paralyzed and only able to get moving again through Him. I could relate to Isaiah 45:3, which says, "I will give you the treasures of darkness and hidden wealth of secret places, so that you may know that it is I, the LORD, the God of Israel, who calls you by your name." We have a hole in our soul that can only be filled by God, and when everything else is stripped away, we can see that more clearly. He is all that remains, all we need. He can never be stripped away from us. I found that God is a forever treasure we will always have, especially in the midst of our darkness.

Struck Down but Not Destroyed

We got up with the alarm clock on Tuesday, December 6, 2016. I remarked to Bob that I wasn't feeling quite right. We proceeded to the bathroom to get ready for our day, and suddenly I felt like I was going to vomit. I sat on the toilet. The last thing I remember was the disconnect in communication between my brain and hand on how to unroll the toilet paper. I woke up sprawled awkwardly on the floor with Bob kneeling over me with his cell phone.

"Who are you calling?" I asked.

"911," he answered.

"What! Why!?" I asked.

"You passed out and I couldn't get you to respond."

"Could we just call Meridith instead? Please just walk me back to bed, and maybe I will feel better," I pleaded.

According to Bob, he was talking to me while I was on the toilet, but I wasn't responding. Then, I lunged backwards a couple of times, let out a long exhale, and fell to the floor. Next came a gurgling sound from my throat. He said he tried to rouse me, but I was unresponsive. He thought he had lost me! That's when he went back to the bedroom to get his phone.

I conceded to the call for emergency help, and soon there were nine paramedics and firefighters standing ominously in our bedroom. I was strapped onto the gurney, rolled out to the ambulance waiting in front of our house, and driven to our hospital. The thing I kept thinking during my ambulance ride was, "I'm sure glad I put on my new pajamas last night."

After a day of tests in the emergency department, an overnight stay for extra precautions, and additional procedures the next day, I was discharged. The tests ruled out all the big stuff—no cancer in the brain, no stroke, no blood clots, no heart problems, no seizures. Since this was my first fainting episode in my life, the doctors assumed it was just a fluke, and nothing to be overly concerned about unless it happened again.

I had only been taking Zoloft for a few days before I had this syncope episode. After that unpleasant experience, we decided to forgo this medication. The Ativan remained on my medication list, as I still had anxiety about sleeping, and it seemed to help. I did not take it every night, just as needed, which was not very often. Sometimes just knowing it is available was enough to calm me down.

I had a follow-up with my oncologist on January 3rd, as to how I was feeling emotionally. I confessed to him that I had stopped taking the antidepressant. He said as long as I was feeling well, that was fine. I was much improved and very thankful for the prayers of many. My oncologist was pleased and didn't need to see me for four months. He reminded me, though, that he was just a phone call away. That was reassuring, but what's even more reassuring is that our awesome God is just a prayer away!

Since May 2016, all my tests and blood work had been "negative" or "normal." This is when negative is good! I remember looking at my medical chart after the smooth, uneventful birth of my first child back in 1986. The OB/GYN had written that I was "unremarkable." My first thought was "How rude, that's not a nice thing to say!" But then I realized that "unremarkable" in medical speak is a positive thing! After having previously been referred to as an enigma and a conundrum, it was refreshing to see the word "normal" on my medical chart.

Even though I still had eight or so years left of hormonal therapy, fairly frequent doctor exams, and continued healing from my cancer treatments, I started to think of myself as a survivor. A survivor, not just from breast cancer but also from its side effects, including depression. And this—all of this—was only possible with God, who never left me—even through complete darkness.

CHAPTER 10

Learning to Live Again

I felt full of life as we walked the legendary Hospital Hill Half-Marathon on June 3rd, 2017. That's exactly how I wanted to celebrate my 57th birthday. I have run or walked many races over the years, but being able to compete in the longest race of my life after a marathon of cancer appointments made this one extra special. "Let's really push it this last mile," Meridith said as we crested the final hill, viewing spectacular downtown Kansas City!

"I've been pushing it the whole race!" I answered. Throwing caution to the wind, though, knowing I was walking with my own private nurse who could resuscitate me if necessary, I pressed on. I focused solely on moving forward one foot then the other, blocked out distractions, and singled in on the cheering crowd and then the finish line! 13.1 miles done in just over three hours. Meridith and I had so much to celebrate—one year prior she was facing at least two brain surgeries and I had just finished aggressive breast cancer treatment. We enjoyed a girl weekend downtown relaxing and recounting our blessings.

Adjusting back to the land of the living was confusing. Changing from fighting for my life to finding how to live again was difficult. After all, one of my cancer doctors said, "Breast cancer is very unforgiving," meaning it can be stubborn and not let your body forget it had cancer. Plus, there's always the chance it could recur. I often felt like a yo-yo: *I'm going to die—now I'm alive! I'm cured and moving on—I think the cancer is back!*

Just as I finally "arrived" (got it in my head to go forward with life), I found myself at the same mammogram and ultrasound center where my cancer was diagnosed. My oncologist was concerned about a tough area near where I had lymph nodes removed, so he wanted it thoroughly checked out. Both tests were done in eerie deja vu, followed by the tortuous wait for answers. I sat near the technician and watched as she communicated via computer with the radiologist. She clicked this picture, then that one, typed something, answered a question or two, then repeated the process. I waited, watched, and prayed as this scenario continued for several minutes. About the time I was convinced the cancer was back, she turned to me and said, "You are free to go. Everything checked out okay." Back to living.

I had been having side effects to my hormonal therapy drug, Femara (letrozole), which my oncologist had switched me to in the fall of 2016. The most difficult side effect was bone and muscle pain. My PCP prescribed Mobic (meloxicam) to combat the pain. Wanting to get to the bottom of the pain, my oncologist orchestrated a test. He had me stop taking Femara for two weeks to see if the pain went away. Then he had me take it again for two additional weeks to see if the pain came back. I felt terrific during the drug holiday and bad again when I resumed the med, so he assumed Femara was the culprit to my pain.

He then switched me to Aromasin (exemestane). I ended up with pain on Aromasin as well. Many weeks later, my oncologist took me off Aromesin and put me back on tamoxifen, my original hormonal therapy drug. Even though research suggests that aromatase inhibitors are more effective against my type of breast cancer, the side effects were grueling to endure. I was having continual bone pain, which had me feeling miserable almost constantly. My only side effect of tamoxifen was hot flashes. While annoying, the hot flashes were much more manageable than the pain.

Why Not Me?

One important part of a cancer-fighter's journey is battle buddies, fellow cancer-fighters who can commiserate, cry, and pray together. One such friend to me was battling glioblastoma. We prayed for healing, both for her and for me. We had sweet fellowship studying Scripture on the phone from Kansas City to Indiana, encouraging and uplifting each other in the Word of God. We kept coming back to the theme of assurance, of Christian hope. "This hope we have as an anchor of the soul, a hope both sure and steadfast" (Hebrews 6:19a). We both clung to this not hopeful but *sure* hope.

Just as I started adjusting to life again I got word that this friend passed away. News like this rocks me to the core and causes me to ask, "Why her and not me?" I miss my friend dearly. While I experienced healing, she lost her life. Did God not answer our prayers? Why was my life spared, but not hers? Sometimes God doesn't give us exactly what we request, but He still answers. God does hear us when we pray. He responds, not necessarily how we ask Him to, but according to His great wisdom.

Knowing that God loves us and is fair, gives us confidence as we wait for answers to prayers. Isaiah 30:18 says, "Therefore the Lord longs to be gracious to you, and therefore He waits on high to have compassion on you.

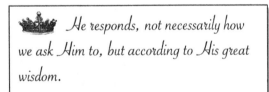

He responds, not necessarily how we ask Him to, but according to His great wisdom.

For the Lord is a God of justice; how blessed are all those who long for Him." His answer is based on these truths: God is gracious, compassionate, and just.

When I was pregnant with our third child, I wanted and prayed for another son. I told God all the reasons it would be best for us to have three boys and no girls. In fact, when the nurses attending me in the delivery room exuberantly exclaimed, "It's a girl!" I was shocked and disappointedly said, "I wanted a boy!" In hindsight, I am so grateful God gave me what

He knew we needed rather than what I thought I wanted! I have so loved having my daughter Meridith. She was physically with us when we got the news I had cancer. She was by my side at the start of treatment. Then, with her nursing knowledge, she has been a constant confidant throughout the whole medical process. I couldn't have foreseen this in my selfish little prayer when she was in my womb, but perhaps one reason God gave Meridith to me was for this specific care I would need and value from a daughter during this difficult time. God is sovereign over us, which brings great comfort to me.

So I ask myself, "Why was my glioblastoma friend's life cut short when mine wasn't?" But then I realized that her life wasn't cut short at all. As I heard one pastor put it, "We bury bodies, not people." We all have an eternity to live; it begins the moment we are conceived. My friend trusted Christ as her Lord and Savior. She was made right with God through the blood of Jesus. So now, though she is absent from the body, she is present with the Lord (2 Corinthians 5:8). God in His great wisdom knew it was the right time to bring her home. I keep thinking of her walking the streets of gold, visiting with saints of old.

Coming face to face with death does make you think about dying. Hebrews 9:27-28 confirms, "And inasmuch as it is appointed for men to die once and after this comes judgment, so Christ also, having been offered once to bear the sins of many, will appear a second time for salvation without reference to sin, to those who eagerly await Him." We will all die once, but we will all also live forever; after this earth we will either go to Heaven or Hell. Those who believed on the Lord Jesus Christ will join Him in Heaven, and those who did not will be eternally separated from Him in Hell. There is only one way to be saved, as Acts 4:12 declares, "And there is salvation in no one else; for there is no other name under heaven that has been given among men by which we must be saved."

There is a difference between knowing *about* God and *knowing* God. Having knowledge about Him or believing Jesus was a good teacher is not enough. We must believe that He died in our place, paying the penalty for our sins. As Jesus Himself put it, "I am the way, the truth, and the life; no one comes to the Father but through me" (John 14:6). This is the only true way to know God. Putting our faith in Christ to save us is the most important decision we can make. Nothing is more crucial than a right relationship with God.

At the start of my cancer battle in 2015, not knowing that exactly one year later she would also be in the war, this is what my battle buddy wrote to me:

"I'm thinking of you daily—often. Your testimony for the Lord is absolutely precious. I don't know what you are going through not having walked in your shoes; I hope that I would have similar strength, courage, and a desire to glorify the Lord Jesus Christ so that others might see His love through me as you have shown."

You did it, dear friend, you showed God's love and shared Christ's salvation to those you encountered as you walked that undesired cancer road! I felt your concern for your medical team as you shared your faith with them, saw you uplifting Christ on your social media posts, heard how you ministered to your family through deed and the Word. Well done, good and faithful servant!

The death of a Christian can be as celebrated as the birth of a baby! After all, we are being born into our new life in Heaven. Of course, I'm sad for me, her family, and loved ones in the meantime, but I'm oh-so-happy for her as she has seen Jesus face to face!

Many friends who have been diagnosed with cancer after me have died, yet I am still here. I continue to lose friends to cancer, but they aren't gone. Our relationship has just changed. If we are saved, we will be reunited again someday and what a great reunion that will be! 1 Corinthians 15:55 asks, "O, death, where is your victory? O death, where is your sting?" Though death will come, it has no lasting power because Jesus Christ defeated death by rising from the grave and extending eternal life to all who trust in Him alone. This world is not our home, we're just passing through. If we are Christians, we are aliens in this world; our citizenship is in Heaven.

Hello, Cancer, My Old Friend

The call came on a Friday evening as we were getting ready for our weekly movie night. Bob had gone to pick up our Redbox selection, when the phone rang. I debated about not answering it, until I noticed the number was my hospital. After the resident identified himself, he said, "Your skin biopsy came back positive." A flood of anxiety and emotion caused my need to pull up a chair and sit down. As he proceeded and said the word "cancer" I thought, *So this is it. This is what the oncologist warned could happen; the cancer is back.*

Turns out it was just pigmented nodular basal cell carcinoma on my back, and a month later was totally excised, but now my dermatologist wanted to see me regularly.

My hospital had a webinar about the psychological effects of a cancer diagnosis. Cancer patients can become overly fearful, thinking their cancer's return is just around every corner. The correct attitude is to be cautious enough to see and feel abnormalities in order to alert your doctors should further testing be needed, but not overly worried to the point of living in fear.

We have to learn to live once more, figuring out how to move on after treatment. When we are diagnosed with cancer, first there's shock, denial, and hoping it isn't true. Next comes acceptance, treatment, attention of medical personnel, cards, and visits from friends. Finally, treatment ends and we are pronounced "cured." Now we have to pick up the pieces of our new life and move on, but we're always thinking in the back of our minds, "When is cancer going to rear its ugly head again?"

But how? Who am I? What now? I am learning that when you finish your active treatment for cancer, it's not over—you can't close the door completely. Once you have cancer, it has you. But it shouldn't be your master.

My PCP said it was time for my second colonoscopy. It was sooner than the normal recommendation, but considered necessary with my cancer risk. The gastroenterologist told me he removed one polyp to be sent in for testing. If it was okay, he would release the results via computer, if cancerous, he would call me. A few days later, I was shaken as I saw a call coming in from the hospital! I answered it, steeling myself for the suspected bad news, but it was just a call to tell us Bob's glasses were ready to be picked up! See, this nerve-wracking feeling never wears off! The removed polyp was precancerous, but slow growing; I will have a repeat colonoscopy in five years.

My hair grew back—enough for regular haircuts.

Psalm 112:7 offers a healthy attitude of the unknown: "He will not fear evil tidings; his heart is steadfast, trusting in the LORD." God proved Himself faithful to me throughout my cancer journey. People would say, "I don't know how you can cope so well with your breast cancer diagnosis and treatment," but God's grace truly was sufficient to meet my needs. Before my diagnosis, I didn't think I could have endured such a trial, but God, in each moment, gave me the grace when I needed it. I wasn't in the trial alone. Many people were raising me up before the throne of grace, and those answers from our Father carried me through. I learned that no matter what happens, we are never alone; God is always walking beside us (or even carrying us).

Is Life Worth Living?

When it first hit me that I had cancer, I secretly wondered if I really wanted to keep living without the femininity of my breasts. Would I still be me? I can say on the other side—yes! Definitely, life has still been worth living. My breasts aren't what made me a woman. It's not our body parts, but our soul that defines us. We are a soul that inhabits a body, not the other way around. Our body dies, but our soul lives on forever.

After I was diagnosed with breast cancer, I saw my oncologist weekly through chemotherapy. Then my oncology visits and lab work became every two weeks, then monthly, then every four months, then twice a year. My daughter was home and accompanied me to my oncology appointment in July of 2019. All blood work was normal, with the exception of slightly low white blood count (chemo caused, and probably permanent).

For months after chemotherapy, radiation, cancer surgeries, and hormonal therapy, I was tired, achy, and fatigued. But in the summer of 2019, I had gotten a renewed sense of energy again, I almost felt like my precancerous self. Therefore, even though a little fearsome to me, it made sense when my oncologist suggested he only needed to see me once a year.

I would be anxious about the possibility of cancer recurrence leading up to and during each oncology appointment, but overall my oncologist had become my security blanket. Knowing I had these frequent visits with my oncologist gave me assurance that my body was getting a thorough check over, reassuring me that the cancer was still at bay. I would walk in the office timid and cautious, but then leave the office with a big sigh of relief knowing the cancer had not returned. Now my oncologist wanted to put more time between our visits. More growth in learning to live again!

CHAPTER 11

God is Still Good

I had been enjoying life for several months, feeling back to my pre-cancer self. It had been over four years since my breast cancer diagnosis. The more time that had passed, the better chances that I had beaten the breast cancer beast for good. I had gotten so used to my daily tamoxifen tablet, that it hardly reminded me that I had been a cancer patient. My cancer was in remission, and many would call me cured. Little symptoms no longer scared me like they did before, so I didn't think much of it when I started having shortness of breath in October of 2019.

I would often walk while talking on the phone with Meridith. I have walked the same beaten path for years. One day while walking and talking, she interrupted me, asking, "Mom, why are you out of breath?"

"I don't know" I replied. We agreed it couldn't be that I was out of shape, since I'd been highly active for several years, fast-walking daily. I was on an uphill slope when she asked this, but I had purposely sought out and walked hills in my daily detailed training.

"You need to call your PCP and get this checked out," she said.

"Oh, Sweetie, it's probably just my allergies kicking in. Let me give it a few weeks to see if it goes away."

Really, I thought, *it's no big deal*. I have dealt with seasonal allergies for years and got used to a runny nose, cough, sore throat, and chest congestion. The shortness of breath, though, was a new symptom, but it wasn't *that* bad. I was fifty-nine now, after all. Maybe this just comes with aging? The shortness of breath was only when I was walking fast, uphill, and talking to someone.

Over the course of the next couple of weeks, Meridith would reiterate all the medical issues that could cause shortness of breath and the necessity of seeing my doctor about it. So, to appease her, I messaged my PCP on October 19th, explaining that I was finding it harder to catch my breath when walking uphill. By this time, I was also having a cough with thick drainage. I continued my message, saying that now I was huffing and puffing while riding my exercise bike and trying to talk at the same time. I concluded with, "I'm not having any other respiratory symptoms, but just wanted to fill you in on how I am feeling."

Soon I heard back from another doctor who was covering for mine, saying I should make an appointment with my PCP to get the shortness of breath checked out. I had hoped my doctor would just respond and say, "Let's order a chest X-ray," or "Thanks for letting me know. We'll keep an eye on it." I didn't really feel like taking the time to make an appointment and then go in to see the doctor. I had just had my six-month checkup on October 7th, anyway, and was ecstatic that nothing was found that needed extra attention. I was wondering if this was all in my head because I was feeling fine when I wasn't walking uphill or exercising and talking at the same time.

Meridith came home the first weekend in November so we could attend her alma mater's homecoming festivities. One of those events was a 5K. We knew we would be slow walking it, as she was still recovering from one of her major hip surgeries. She had to stop after mile one, so she told me to do mile two alone. Then we would finish mile three together. I was feeling great, so I decided to run the second mile.

Then my lips went numb, and I thought I was going to pass out. I stopped and found Meridith.

"Mom, no more waiting," she said. "You need to see your doctor about this."

I was able to get in to my PCP's NP on November 11th. She wanted to check out my heart as well as my lungs. That day I had an EKG and Chest X-ray. Those results were both normal. The NP also ordered other tests that were scheduled as soon as they were approved and at first availability.

On November 22nd, I had a Treadmill Exercise Echocardiogram W/2-D + Doppler Echo. My heart tested out fine. The NP said the test looked great.

Meridith was home again for Thanksgiving, and I still wasn't improving. After additional urging, from Mom-Meridith, I contacted my medical team again on November 25th, explaining that, in fact, the shortness of breath was worse, and I had to walk slower than my thirteen-and-a-half-minute mile pace. I was also getting out of breath bending over and when talking. I was having coughing spells daily. My PCP's NP responded back with an order for a D-Dimer blood test, which I had drawn on November 27th. The D-Dimer was negative, which ruled out blood clots or pulmonary embolism. Since I wasn't feeling any better, the NP put in a referral for me to see a pulmonologist (lung doctor). I took the first available appointment, February 3rd.

On December 4th I had a Complete Pulmonary Function Test. The NP got the results to me that same day with the comments, "Your pulmonary function testing is normal. This essentially rules out something like asthma or COPD."

I sent another message to my PCP's NP that evening, asking if there was anything else they could do to ease my symptoms since I had a long wait until the appointment with the pulmonologist. I was still out of breath when talking and walking. If I was walking uphill and talking, I had to stop talking; otherwise, I felt like I would pass out. Even one flight of stairs or bending over caused me to huff and puff. She decided to prescribe an inhaler, which I was glad to try, especially when exercising.

On December 23rd, I messaged my NP again with an update. At this time, I had been using the inhaler for almost two weeks. Initially, it seemed to make my coughing more productive. I kept wanting to say it was helping with the shortness of breath when walking, but I still felt like I was going to pass out going uphill while talking and walking. Meridith watched me use the inhaler to make sure I was operating it correctly. She said I should feel relief from it immediately, but that wasn't happening. The shortness of breath when bending over continued, and sometimes it bothered me while sitting and crossing my arms over my chest. I was coughing a lot more, especially when first waking up.

In my research I read that tamoxifen could cause shortness of breath—maybe this was my problem, I wondered? I was beginning to think I needed to bring my oncologist into our discussion. At this point I had been Googling reasons for shortness of breath. Of course, cancer was one possible cause, but I really didn't think that was what was going on with me. I just thought my oncologist would be an additional mind to help solve my breathing problem.

On December 30th, I received a message from my NP asking if I was still having respiratory issues and wondering if the symptoms had gotten worse. She wanted me to come in for a follow-up visit.

I saw her on January 2nd, and she decided a Chest CT scan would be prudent, as the pulmonologist would probably want one. Doing the CT before the appointment would give him the data ahead of time. "Do you think we should let my oncologist know?" I asked.

She said yes, and she would send him my recent office visit notes and update him on all my symptoms and test results. I scheduled the Chest CT scan before I left the office, taking the first available—January 17th.

How Can This Be?

Bob's office was moving to a four-day work week, and January 17th was his first Friday off. It also coincided with Restaurant Week in our city. This is an annual event where various restaurants feature a specific menu at a special price, giving some of their proceeds to charity. This is a win-win situation—the restaurants get people into their establishments during a slow season, and customers get a great deal on fabulous food. We booked an early reservation on that Friday evening at a nice steak house that was conveniently situated between our home and the hospital. Therefore, by God's providence, Bob went with me to the CT scan when otherwise I probably would have gone alone.

They got me in ahead of schedule for the Chest CT scan, so I was finished too early for us to head to the restaurant. We decided to sit in the waiting room for a bit. Bob had a book to read. I opened my phone to work on this book (chapter 1, to be exact). Ominous feelings swirled around me as I sat there writing about my cancer journey in the hospital where I had been diagnosed four and a half years earlier. I reminded myself these were just emotions I was reliving, since I was actively writing about those past experiences.

Soon it was time to head to the restaurant. While getting in the car, my phone rang. Seeing it was coming from the hospital, I answered it. "Maybe they need me to come back in and repeat an image for the CT," I thought.

"Camy," my PCP said. "Where are you?"

"We are just leaving the hospital," I replied.

"Are you alone?" she asked. "No, Bob is here. Let me put you on speaker," I replied as we both sat down and buckled our seat belts.

My PCP proceeded to explain the startling and unexpected results from my just-finished "abnormal" Chest CT scan. "I'm afraid I don't have good news to relay from your Chest CT." She paused, then gingerly continued, "I am so sorry. Your CT shows innumerable nodules throughout both lungs, which look like cancer." She took a breath then continued, "The CT also shows possible lymph node involvement as well as probable cancer in the liver."

It appeared as though my cancer had returned—with a vengeance.

Obviously emotionally affected herself, my PCP said, "I am so sorry. No wonder you're having trouble breathing."

After we thanked her for letting us know what was going on in my body, she went on to say, "I am 100% shocked with the results of the CT. This is unusual, atypical, and not at all what I was expecting to see."

My PCP stayed on the phone as long as we needed her to repeat what she had already said and to answer any questions we had, also saying she would release the CT report so we could read it ourselves. "I'm sorry to have to be the bearer of bad news, but I knew if I were in your shoes, I would want this news as soon as it was discovered."

She said she would reach out to my oncologist to determine the next steps, "I'm sure you will hear from him soon. Unfortunately, our offices are closed Monday for Martin Luther King Jr. Day. Hang in there," she added warmly before hanging up.

What moments before had been surreal, now became real as we processed the foreboding news of probable metastatic cancer. Honestly, I felt the same as my PCP—total shock. I was truly, not at all expecting the news to be cancer. I assumed I was having exercise-induced asthma, or something fixable like that. I turned to Bob and with tears in my eyes said, "I am so sorry." I had witnessed that cancer is often harder on the family members than the patient. I knew this meant stage four, terminal.

My cancer would no longer be curable.

Bob led us in a prayer to God, thanking Him for a diagnosis to my shortness of breath, although definitely not the answer we were hoping for. He also prayed for strength, guidance, and help as we headed down this cancer road once again.

When he said, "amen," I said, "Let's go to dinner," though I was feeling more hungry for answers than for food. We sat there eating a tasty steak dinner, complete with crème brûlée, all the while talking about how our world had just been turned upside down again.

Meridith reached out to see how my scan had gone. I couldn't yet talk about it, so I just texted to her, "Not good. I will forward to you the scan results."

Despite the terrible news, we were grateful my PCP contacted us as soon as she found out. I was impressed at how quickly we got the results from the scan. My CT finished at 2:52 PM, the radiologist called the NP at 3:17, and the findings were finalized at 3:23. We received the phone call from my PCP at 3:34.

My CT results read:

1. Development of innumerable bilateral pulmonary nodules and areas of interlobular septal thickening, most compatible with pulmonary metastatic disease and lymphangitic carcinomatosis.
2. Development of mild thoracic lymphadenopathy, compatible with nodal metastases.
3. Development of multiple ill-defined hypoattenuating hepatic lesions, most compatible with hepatic metastases.

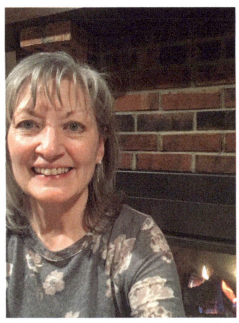

I snapped this picture during an evening of many tears after my oncologist confirmed my cancer was back.

Meridith wrote the following letter on January 23rd, two days after my oncologist confirmed that my cancer had returned. Her letter captures how we all felt:

Cancer,

I was ecstatic at the news that we had beaten you. The surgery, chemotherapy, radiation and hormonal therapy had done its job taming you. This victory meant mom could be promoted to yearly oncology appointments and labs rather than facing her fear of you every few months. If I ever see you again, it will be too soon!

This past November, I proofread mom's book about her experience fighting you, re-living all the emotions we felt upon hearing you had invaded her body. But these memories left me feeling empowered because you were a thing of the past. Your attack shattered our world, yet through it, we grew closer as a family and stronger in our faith in Christ.

When mom's breathing trouble began this past fall, anxiety flooded me at the thought that you could be emerging again. But an X-ray, which revealed no tumors, squelched that fear. Something else, less scary than cancer, was plaguing her.

Metastasis. Carcinoma.

My heart plummeted to my toes upon reading these words in mom's chest CT results. Innumerable nodules throughout the liver and lungs. Was this really mom's scan, or had there been a mix-up between patients? Tears streamed down my face, my mind spinning with the myriad of tests, treatment and heartache that now loomed ahead.

Cancer, I'm not ready to face you again. Mom doesn't deserve to endure you again. It wasn't supposed to happen this way!

Cancer, this was supposed to be the year mom and I waved goodbye to our roller-coaster health struggles, accomplishing milestones together such as a 60-mile breast cancer walk. Though you've upended our dreams, we won't let you steal our passion for life. We will seize every moment, living it to the fullest, holding closely the things that are most precious.

– Meridith

Here We Go Again

Sure enough, on Tuesday, January 21st at 8 AM, my oncologist's nurse called. Could I come in for labs at 2:30 and an appointment with the oncologist at 3? Absolutely!

My oncologist wanted me to fill him in on what had happened medically since he had seen me when everything appeared fine on July 30, 2019. He said he was home when he got the news from my PCP about my abnormal CT scan and was surprised at how the cancer presented itself. He concurred with everything my PCP and NP had done. Being an oncologist, he said he probably would have done the Chest CT scan sooner, but my PCP and NP certainly followed protocol. He did say he didn't think we had lost any ground as far as treatment went.

My oncologist confirmed what we already suspected, this time my cancer was treatable, but not curable. If breast cancer spreads to another part of the body, it is called advanced, metastatic, or stage four breast cancer. At this stage the cancer cannot be cured. I was relieved my oncologist wanted to help me fight, as I was afraid my cancer had spread too far for any treatment.

My doctor went into great detail outlining the variable cancer scenarios, told us the tests and procedures he would order for me now and later. He then explained the different options available to treat my cancer. He paused, at one point, looked up, and said, "Did you get that?"

"Uh, no," I replied, "but I like how your brain works!" Although much of what my oncologist said went over my head, I was reassured knowing he had my best interest in mind and was going to attack this cancer with every arsenal he had at his disposal.

He also said that if all conventional options for me fail, we would then try clinical trials. He did say if treatment became too difficult on my body, we'd have to switch to comfort care. He told us that typically a survivor in my situation has three to four years to live.

The reason my cancer didn't show up on the November X-ray was because the tumors in the lungs were so small. It is his belief that the cancer is what had caused the shortness of breath from the beginning.

A biopsy of my liver was scheduled to confirm that this was metastatic *breast* cancer and not a new cancer. This biopsy would also determine the type of chemotherapy I would receive as well as if I would need hormonal therapy or immunotherapy. Surgery and radiation were not indicated this time around due to the small size and scattering of the tumors. An Abdominal/Pelvic CT scan and a Whole Body Bone Scan were scheduled to determine if there was cancer anywhere else.

A CA-27.29 (Tumor Marker) blood test was done on January 21st. My value measured at 2,233 U/mL; normal is <=38 U/mL. This is a test primarily used to monitor stage four metastatic breast cancer. It can show the progression of cancer; increasing values correspond with advancing disease. The test is also useful to tell if treatment is working; lower values correspond with a positive treatment response.

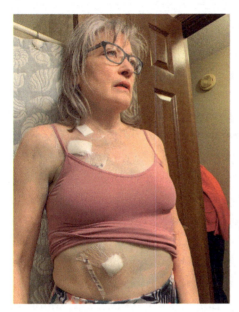

Port placement and liver biopsy.

My port placement and liver biopsy went off fairly easily on January 27th. An added surprise was bumping into my PCP's nurse while checking in; what a comfort it was to get a pre-surgery hug from her!

The doctors, techs, and nurses communicated with me throughout the two procedures, as they used conscious sedation, so I was alert and communicative. The insertion of the port was painless. This is exactly the same type of port I had four and a half years ago, only this time it was inserted on the other side of my upper chest.

There was some pain with the biopsy, but the swiftness of the procedure made it bearable. Percutaneous liver biopsy is a procedure in which a tiny sample of the liver tissue is taken using a needle inserted through the skin and into the liver, guided by ultrasound. The procedure lasted less than one hour. It was interesting to be awake during this process, listening and being a part of the conversations amongst the physicians, nurses, and other medical personnel in the operating room. I was intrigued looking around the operating room at all the equipment and many people doing their respective duties. I told myself to rest in the arms of Jesus. I kept thanking God that my new cancer diagnosis hadn't taken *Him* by surprise.

I was wheeled back to recovery and had a two- to four-hour monitoring period before I was allowed to return home, as extra bleeding can occur with the liver biopsy procedure.

> *I kept thanking God that my new cancer diagnosis hadn't taken Him by surprise.*

After two hours, Bob went to get the car, and I started getting dressed. All of the sudden, I felt like I was going to faint and throw up. I was in the bathroom, and a nurse was right outside the door. I told her how I felt, and she immediately called for reinforcements, sat me in a wheelchair, and took me back to a bed. They reattached the many vital sign paraphernalia. My systolic blood pressure had dropped to 60 and my heart rate was an alarming 40. They started IV fluids, I rested a bit, then ate a sandwich. We were on our way home after another three hours of monitoring, doctor visits, and proving I could walk around the room safely.

Leaving the hospital that day, Bob and I both had mounting foreboding, familiar, yucky feelings about the continuing treatment process of my cancer.

Stronger and More Empowered

When I received my original breast cancer diagnosis in June of 2015, I remember all too well feeling so completely devastated and scared that Bob and Meridith had to take over scheduling all my appointments, talking to doctors for me, and even responding to family and friends on my behalf. This time around, however, I felt stronger emotionally from my previous experience with cancer and better armed for the battle. I chose to rely on truth in God's word as in Isaiah 41:13: "For I am the LORD your God, who upholds your right hand, who says to you, 'Do not fear, I will help you.'" I advocated with medical scheduling to get my port placed just ten days after the first news of cancer's return. I was determined and eager to get my treatment started as soon as possible and attack this alien that had taken up residence in my body once again. I phoned Meridith and said, "You taught me well."

Bob and I met with my oncologist's new NP on January 30th. I liked her from the start of our hour-long meeting. Then, when she told me we share a middle name, there was an instant bond between us. How many people do you know who have the middle name Adele?!

She was very thorough at explaining details and side effects of Abraxane, the intravenous chemotherapy I would be getting three times a month. She said this chemo is usually easier on the body than the three kinds I had in 2015. The NP also gave us the heartening news that Abraxane could decrease my coughing and shortness of breath.

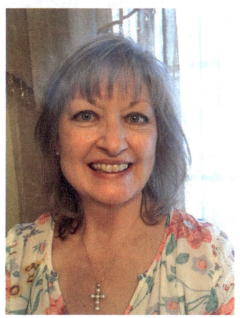

Finally, my hair is long enough to feel "like me" again.

I was disheartened to find out that I would be losing my hair once again. That made me especially sad, as it had just grown to my preferred length and my beautician had recently found a style I really liked! My hair was a part of me that I had a good healthy image of; I genuinely liked my hair. All my life I've received compliments on my hair and felt it was part of who I was. I had grown fond of my new, natural gray color and was delighted that it was long enough to wear in a ponytail again. I had hair I loved before my first cancer diagnosis, then lost it. I once again had hair that I loved and now would lose it too, and this time I might never get it back.

The results from my liver biopsy confirmed that I had stage four metastatic breast cancer and not a new cancer. My markers remained ER/PR positive and HER2 negative. Based on these results, the plan would be at least six months of Abraxane, then hormonal therapy Faslodex (a literal pain-in-the-butt shot, one in each buttock every four weeks), plus a cdk4/6 inhibitor.

The next day Bob accompanied me to my (second) first chemotherapy session. It was eerie entering the infusion room again. A flood of memories came back from the times I spent there almost five years ago. But, the hope that is given from the nurses and seen in patients is inspiring. Many patients were upbeat regardless of their diagnosis, encouraging others to fully enjoy whatever time they have left. The medical professionals continued to mention the many advances and new cancer treatments constantly becoming available. My infusion was painless, and we were on our way home a couple of hours later.

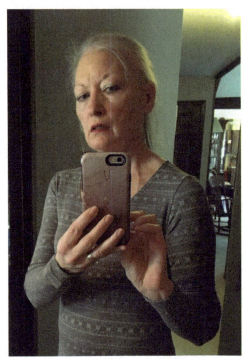

Losing my hair—a second time.

I felt a little icky that first evening, but not nearly as bad as before.

I went to bed grateful to God, that only two weeks since the first inkling that my cancer was back, I was already receiving treatment to fight it.

More Tests and Results

On February 11th, I had an Abdominal/Pelvic CT Scan and Full Body Bone Scan. An RN accessed my port. Then a tech gave me a calcium injection that needed three hours to run its course before the bone scan could be done. They completed the CT scan and then sent us out to wait in the lobby for the calcium to be absorbed into my bones.

To pass the time during our long wait, I decided to work on emails. Upon opening my email app, I immediately noticed a new test result had been posted to my medical chart. I turned to Bob while logging in and said, "It must be good news; otherwise, my oncologist would have called before releasing the results." We opened the test and read this message from him:

> Camy,
>
> The CT scan shows cancer in the liver and surrounding lymph nodes. There may be some cancer in the peritoneal space (having to do with the tissue that lines the abdominal wall and pelvic cavity) as well. This is uncertain. This does not change management currently, but when we rescan, we will know what we started with.
> -GC

Next, we read the full report for ourselves, which was daunting. It's difficult to read things like this about your own body. We were both somewhat discouraged, and I was getting scared of the magnitude of the cancer spread.

I felt like my body was betraying me. I could relate to Psalm 73:26: "My flesh and my heart may fail, but God is the strength of my heart and my portion forever." I reminded myself that God would be with me no matter what the news.

I consulted Meridith, my personal RN, giving her the full report to read. She calmed us down, saying "Essentially the CT scan shows what we already knew." My breast cancer had metastasized to my lungs, liver and lymph nodes. She continued, "The new thing is possible cancer in the peritoneaum."

The bone scan went off as planned. The tech told me that my hospital was the second in the nation to get the sophisticated machine she used on me for this test.

After arriving home, I received an email that my bone scan results were available. I steeled myself as I opened that report:

Camy,

There is no obvious cancer in the bones.
-GC

As the day ended, Bob and I both felt weary, but still grateful. It was, mentally, a yo-yo day. I assumed good news when I saw my CT results posted, then nervous when reading their content showing more cancer. This caused me to be even more worried about the possibility of cancer in my bones, but then when that news came back clear, I felt elated.

Losses and Gains

As I've said before, I've never been afraid of getting cancer, but I've always been afraid of drowning. With the cancer metastasized to my lungs, it looks like I *will* die of drowning after all. Yet, I know I will not be alone. As Isaiah 43:2a says, "When you pass through the waters, I will be with you; and through the rivers, they will not overflow you."

People ask me how I have such great faith. It's not my faith that is big, but rather that my faith is in a big *God*. In fact, sometimes, in those scary or alone times, my faith feels very small. Then I remember *He is able*. My hope is in God, not my circumstances. With God, the possibilities are better than we could ever imagine.

> ♛ *My hope is in God, not my circumstances. With God, the possibilities are better than we could ever imagine.*

As I thought about this metastatic diagnosis, Psalm 124:8 gave me great comfort: "Our help is in the name of the LORD, Who made heaven and earth." Our God created the heavens and the earth from nothing. Surely, He has the power to help me again in my cancer battle. Not only did God create the heavens and earth, but He created me as well. God is the source of my life as stated in Acts 17:24-25, "The God who made the world and all things in it, since He is Lord of heaven and earth, does not dwell in temples made with hands; nor is He served by human hands, as though He needed anything, since He Himself gives to all people life and breath and all things." God formed my body and caused me to breathe; it is His breath in my lungs.

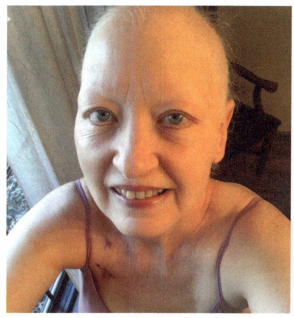
Even if it doesn't look good to me, I can trust whatever God sends my way.

Romans 8:28 says, "And we know that God causes all things to work together for good to those who love God, to those who are called according to His purpose." Was I going to look at this metastatic diagnosis as something good from God? When first diagnosed with breast cancer in June of 2015, I was struck with all I was losing. Looking back from the present vantage point, I can see so many more gains than losses. It all boils down to the right perspective, changing thinking from temporal to eternal.

I often remind myself of two truths: God is sovereign, and God is good. Since God is sovereign, He has everything under control, even my cancer. Since God is good, I can trust everything He sends my way, even if it doesn't look good to me.

As one of my Navy son's shipmates said, "No matter what, God has the final diagnosis."

CHAPTER 12

Even Though I Walk Through the Valley of the Shadow of Death

Same, But Different

I've been down this road before. I went through testing to accurately diagnose my cancer, just as I had the first time. We identified where the cancer was, what type it was, and measured it. We were anxious as we waited for results—how far had it spread? We decided on a treatment plan, started treatment, continued to test to see how effective the treatment was, then adjusted accordingly. All this I had done before. This time, however, there was one glaringly notable difference. This time there was no cure. This time there was only treatment. This time all this treatment is not meant to save my life, but merely prolong it. My body is failing; anything more we can get from it will just be a bonus. My disease is at the fatal stage.

I went bald like last time, but this time I wondered if that was the last time I would ever have hair. Will I live long enough for it to grow out again? Will I feel my hair blow in the wind? Will it grow long enough to tie into a pony tail again? Will I die bald?

Last time, when pain or uncomfortableness from symptoms or treatment came, I used to weigh the harmful side effects of drug intervention, often deciding to endure the pain rather than risk my body with future problems from the side effects. Now, I'm not so against drugs. I most likely won't live long enough to experience the negative long-term effects of them on my body.

Last time, I got my port removed right away when I had my mastectomy. This time my oncologist said to leave my port in after my IV chemotherapy. With constant research, there might be another treatment or test we'd need the port for. I'm guessing I'll go to my grave with this power port still in my body.

Last time, I was eager for cancer treatment to end so I could get on with my life. This time I don't want treatment to end. The end of my treatment will likely usher in the end of my life.

Last time, when Meridith came to stay with me during my mastectomy and reconstruction surgeries, we eagerly talked about me getting well and the fun things we would do together after treatment. This time she has checked with her nurse manager about requesting time off through the Family and Medical Leave Act (FMLA), making plans to be my Hospice nurse if that need is there at the end of my life.

Last time, I was defeating cancer. Now it is defeating me.

Psalm 94:19 says, "When my anxious thoughts multiply within me, your consolations delight my soul." Regularly I have anxious thoughts. I use God as my sounding board. I tell Him my woes, sorrows, fears, and disappointments. I am uplifted by the words in the Bible and God's constant consistency in following through with what He promises. Therefore, I will continue this road with resolve to follow the path He has called me to, knowing He is here with me and He will keep me safe in His arms to the end of my life. There's no cure for my cancer, but I still have a life to live.

I saw my plastic surgeon a few weeks after my metastatic diagnosis. He told me the most important things I could do are to hang on to hope and keep the faith. Many have said it's important for me to stay positive, keep living, continue healthy habits, and thank God for the good news! After all, I am still alive; I need to keep living!

I was adamant at keeping up with my walking, even at a slower pace, as my medical team said being in good shape would help me fight the cancer. I also rode my exercise bike and added arm weights to my work out. I joined a yoga class, which is offered by a nonprofit organization sponsored by my hospital for people affected by chronic or serious illnesses. I like this optimistic quote from their webpage, "We can't change your situation. But we can help you change the way you respond to it."

I have weepy moments. To be honest, I broke down and cried while writing this chapter. A friend told me, "It's normal to be sad when sad things happen." Feeling sad isn't wrong.

My medical team thought it would be good for me to have an appointment with their cancer psychologist.

Here's some wisdom I gleaned from him:
- "You can't and shouldn't protect your family from the emotions they have concerning your diagnosis." When I was diagnosed with cancer this second time, I apologized to my family for putting them through this again. I need to release them to freely undergo and express their feelings.
- "Being open and connecting with people is important." I have shared my fears and sorrows with many family members and friends. It is therapeutic for me to talk to people and I am grateful to those not afraid to hear my sufferings or see my tears.
- "It's helpful to talk about how we feel." Sometimes our talking is thinking out loud and a good way to work through a problem.

- "It's good to be honest about my future." Being allowed to talk about my death and plans at the end exposes the elephant in the room. I appreciate that my family and friends have given me the freedom to do so.
- "Reprioritizing is important." Now that I know I have less time on this earth than I would have thought, how should I best spend it? Wanting to live life well these last three to four years is easy to say, but hard to do.
- "The path we're on might not be the one we planned or expected, but be willing to experience both the good and bad times." So often we try to get rid of the bad times rather than experience them. Our worst times can, surprisingly, turn into the best times. Every difficulty is a possibility.
- "You need to believe your family will be okay too." I hate to think of the pain my family might experience when I die. But God is faithful; He will be there for them after I die as He has been here for me as I'm dying.
- "Your legacy isn't defined by the very last days of your life." I worry about my grandkids watching me die, but I need to remember that won't be their only memory of me.

Psalm 145:17 says, "The LORD is righteous in all His ways and kind in all His deeds." I know that God has the power to heal me, but if He chooses not to, He is still worthy of our praise. He is the One True God, and that is reason enough to praise Him. The fact that He sent His Son, Jesus, who through His blood offered us cleansing of our sins and a home in Heaven is another reason to praise God. After I'm gone, my family can thank God that I am well and at home with Jesus. God's ways are always right and He is always kind.

I Will Fear No Evil, for YOU Are with Me

Three to four years to live? I now know I will probably die of cancer. I'll be fighting this the rest of my life. I am terminal. But we are all terminal—mine is just staring me in the face. Any day could be our last—cancer or no cancer. We don't know when our time on this earth will end. James 4:14 says, "Yet you do not know what your life will be like tomorrow. You are just a vapor that appears for a little while and then vanishes away." I'm not afraid to die. To a Christian, death is now a rebirth—like baptism. Death is no longer to be feared. It is our victory. We can be more than conquerors, overwhelmingly victorious, if we succumb to cancer and die, because even death has no power over us. If we die in Christ, we truly live.

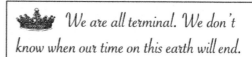

We are all terminal. We don't know when our time on this earth will end.

If we die in Christ we truly live.

There are plans to be made. I'm thinking I should be cleaning, sorting, and throwing stuff away, so my family won't have to do that when I'm gone. Bob and I have picked out our burial place; this isn't long-range planning now, but a necessity. What about funeral plans? I guess I have a few thoughts on that, but, really, I feel that is more for those left behind. I would like to be buried before a memorial service though. I'd really rather my funeral be called a celebration. I won't be there anymore; I'll be home with Jesus.

I do think of the things I'll miss, like another daughter-in-law or son-in-law, watching my grandchildren grow up, more grand babies, growing old with my husband, spending time with family. It makes me sad. I'm tempted to think as each holiday comes and goes, "Will this be my last?" Instead, I remind myself to embrace the moment. Enjoy each day, as Psalm 118:24 says, "This is the day which the LORD has made; let us rejoice and be glad in it." Heaven will be way better than anything I might miss on this earth.

The biggest thing I learned from the first time I had cancer was that God is trustworthy! Our problems do not go away because we have Jesus in our lives, but we will never have to face or solve them on our own.

Every Christian has this hope from Romans 8:38–39: "For I am convinced that neither death, nor life, nor angels, nor principalities, nor things present, nor things to come, nor powers, nor height, nor depth, nor any other created thing, will be able to separate us from the love of God, which is in Christ Jesus or Lord." This doesn't mean we are kept from tragedies, but that God will be with us in them. We can face our fears because God is for us and is with us. We don't have a promise that we'll be pain free or won't get cancer. But, no matter what our struggle is, God will always be there with us. Now nothing can separate us from God, not even cancer. And, even if we get a terminal cancer diagnosis, God is still with us. Even if we die from cancer, God has never left us; we are home with Him. Hallelujah!

Colossians 3:15 says, "Let the peace of Christ rule in your hearts, to which indeed you were called in one body; and be thankful." We need peace *with* God (by becoming a believer in the Lord Jesus Christ) before we can have the peace *of* God in our lives. John 16:33 says, "These things I have spoken to you, so that in Me you may have peace. In the world you have tribulation, but take courage; I have overcome the world." Peace isn't the absence of turmoil, but having the confidence that the Prince of Peace will help us as we go through crises. Let Christ's peace control your heart.

I will fear no evil *because* God is and will be with me. As Psalm 34:4 says, "I sought the LORD, and He answered me, and delivered me from all my fears." The way He delivered me from my fear of dying is the assurance that He will be with me no matter what happens. Psalm 34 goes on to say in verse 18, "The LORD is near to the brokenhearted and saves those who are crushed in spirit." He's got this!

As dark, dismal, and scary the valley can seem at times, and as I ponder that I have received the death sentence, I know I have no reason to fear. I can confidently rest assured in the unwavering truths of the Bible. On the other side is glorious Heaven and I know God will guide and sustain me, walking beside me all the way home. He will get me safely there. It's like 2 Corinthians 4:16–18 says, "Therefore we do not lose heart, but though our outer man is decaying, yet our inner man is being renewed day by day. For momentary, light affliction is producing for us an eternal weight of glory far beyond all comparison, while we look not at the things which are seen, but at the things which are not seen; for the things which are seen are temporal, but the things which are not seen are eternal." As I watch and feel my body die, my spirit is alive and I still have much hope. This temporary difficult road I'm traveling will give way to true life in Heaven with Christ, forever and ever.

God is with me now as I fight this cancer. He will be with my family and friends as they suffer along with me. He will continue to be with us when the time comes for my body to give up the fight. I know my family will be by my side offering comfort and hope until the end. And when I can't see or hear them anymore, I know my Savior God will be with me in the transition from this world to the next. His word promises that He will never leave me.

I have this confidence in death not because of anything I've done, but because of what God did for me. All I did was believe as it says in John 11:25, "Jesus said to her, 'I am the resurrection and the life; he who believes in Me will live even if he dies.'" If you're not a believer yet, I beg you to believe on the Lord Jesus Christ before it is too late. It is just as simple as it sounds. Simple, but not especially easy, as it requires changing your belief system, turning away from what you have followed in the past and truly believing what God in the Bible states as truth. "Believe in the Lord Jesus, and you will be saved" (Acts 16:31a).

Some people think they can get to Heaven by just being good, but that isn't good enough! We must come to God His way. He must be the first in our lives, not just part of our lives. My pastor asked, "Are you just living your life with a little Jesus thrown in?"

We need to follow the truth in God's Word—not "your" truth or "my" truth but *the* truth as Psalm 43:3a says, "O send out Your light and Your truth, let them lead me." There is just *one* way as John 14:6 simply states,

"Jesus said to him, 'I am the way, and the truth, and the life; no one comes to the Father but through Me.'"

I used to think people were arrogant when they said they were sure they were going to Heaven when they die. "How do they know they've been good enough? Can't only God judge that?" I wondered. Then I learned from the Bible it's not our works that save us. It's Jesus' work on the cross.

What we are living now on this earth is just pre-life. After we die, we will live forever. If we are right with Christ, we will truly live. The result of not receiving Christ as our Lord and Savior means living an eternity of torment in Hell. Mark 9:48-49 vividly describes it this way: "where their worm does not die, and the fire is not quenched. For everyone will be salted with fire." My study Bible notes go on to explain that just as salt preserves, everyone who enters Hell will be preserved through an eternity of torment.[2] Mark 1:15 urges, "The time is fulfilled, and the kingdom of God is at hand; repent and believe in the gospel." Our life is like a vapor—**here today, gone tomorrow** (James 4:14)! You might not have tomorrow so please heed the advice of Hebrews 4:7a, "Today if you hear His voice, do not harden your hearts."

It's a New Chapter, Not the Epilogue

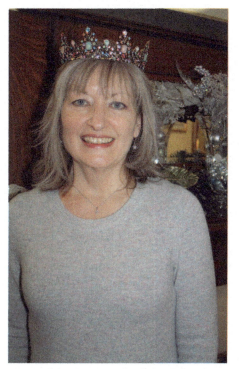

When I got the metastatic terminal diagnosis, I had just finished my book, which had ten chapters. I then wrote an epilogue in my head. Shortly thereafter, I heard a radio pastor say, "How well we handle our losses is a new chapter, not the epilogue." At the same time, my son Thomas encouraged me to add two more chapters instead of an epilogue. An epilogue is the final commentary about the end of a story. But I didn't *know* the end of my story... until my cancer came back. God is writing my story, and He gave me two more chapters. These two chapters are the crown. All the lessons I had learned came to a head. The gift He gave me in this terminal diagnosis—everything I gained through the losses—provides me with a gift I can give back to Him (a crown I can lay down at His feet).

Notes

1. Burnham, Gracia. *In the Presence of My Enemies*. Wheaton: Tyndale House Publishers, 2003.
2. Ryrie, Charles C. *Ryrie Study Bible* NASB. Chicago: Moody Press, Chicago, 1978.

APPENDIX A

CANCER TIMELINE

2015

- January 10 — Robert discovers a lump in my right breast.
- January 21 — Appointment with PCP concerning lump.
- January 27 — Diagnostic Mammogram and Sonogram of right breast.
- January 29 — Mammogram "benign calcifications," Sonogram "negative." Told to, "Return in one year."
- June 4 — Scary return appointment with PCP, as lump had grown.
- June 5 — Nightmarish Diagnostic Mammogram and Sonogram.
- June 9 — First appointment with breast surgeon at my NCI hospital. (All subsequent appointments at NCI hospital).
- June 15 — Repeat Diagnostic Mammogram and Sonogram. Biopsies of breast, skin, and lymph nodes. Radiologist: "It's highly likely this is cancer."
- June 17 — Diagnosis with Breast Surgeon: "Yes, you have breast cancer, but it's treatable." "Invasive ductal carcinoma, nuclear grade 3, histologic grade 2. Malignant cell groups in dermis, lymph node metastatic ductal carcinoma, ER+, PR+, Her2/neu-, Ki-67 borderline, tumor size: 2-5 cm."
- June 22 — Labs and first appointment with oncologist, Genetic study blood draw.
- June 23 — Breast MRI.
- June 26 — Echocardiogram, Chemotherapy education with oncology, Labs.
- June 29 — Power Port Placement.
- July 1 — Torso PET scan.
- July 2 — Labs, Checkup with oncologist, Chemo #1 (Adriamycin & Cytoxan).

- July 3 — Neulasta shot.
- July 9 — Labs, Checkup with oncology.
- July 13 — Wig fitting and purchase.
- July 16 — Labs, Checkup with oncologist, Chemo #2 (Adriamycin & Cytoxan).
- July 17 — Neulasta shot.
- July 19 — Head shaving as hair was falling out profusely.
- July 23 — Labs, Visit with oncology nurse.
- July 30 — Labs, Checkup with oncologist, Chemo #3 (Adriamycin & Cytoxan), Breast reconstruction seminar.
- July 31 — Neulasta shot.
- August 5 — Uterine Sonogram.
- August 6 — Labs.
- August 13 — Labs, Checkup with oncologist, Chemo #4 (Adriamycin & Cytoxan).
- August 14 — Neulasta Shot.
- August 20 — Labs.
- August 27 — Labs, Checkup with oncologist, Chemo #5 (Taxol). Appointment with breast surgeon.
- September 10 — Labs, Checkup with oncologist, Chemo #6 (Taxol).
- September 13 — Race for the Cure.
- September 24 — Labs, Checkup with oncologist, Chemo #7 (Taxol).
- October 7 — Lymphedema prevention education.
- October 8 — Labs, Checkup with oncologist, Last chemo (Taxol).
- October 12 — Checkup with breast surgeon, First appointment with plastic surgeon.
- November 4 — First appointment with radiation oncologist. Pre-Op labs, Echocardiogram and EKG.
- November 11 — Double Mastectomy Surgery. Pathology report: "Invasive ductal carcinoma, intermediate grade, nuclear grade 3, metastatic to 4 of 11 lymph nodes," Acellular dermal matrix and tissue expanders inserted.
- November 16 — Post-Op with plastic surgeon to check skin and incision healing.
- November 23 — No infection or wounds, Tissue expansion begins.
- November 30 — Tissue expansion with plastic surgeon.
- December 1 — Follow-up with breast surgeon.
- December 3 — Labs, Checkup with oncologist.
- December 7 — Tissue expansion with plastic surgeon.

- December 14 — Tissue expansion with plastic surgeon.
- December 21 — Checkup with plastic surgeon.

2016

- January 4 — Checkup with plastic surgeon.
- January 5 — Appointment with radiation oncologist, Radiation Simulation.
- January 11 — Chest X-ray, Appointment with radiation oncologist (Follow-up chest X-rays and radiation oncologist checkups: January 19, 25, February 1, 9, 16, 22.)
- January 11–February 24 — Thirty radiation treatments "linear accelerator-right chest wall."
- February 25 — Started taking Nolvadex.
- February 1 — Checkup with plastic surgeon.
- February 4 — Labs, Checkup with oncologist.
- February 16 — Brain CT scan.
- February 25 — First haircut since hair grew back.
- February 29 — Checkup with plastic surgeon.
- March 10 — Lymphedema prevention follow-up.
- March 23 — Checkup with radiation oncologist.
- March 31 — Last appointment with breast surgeon, as she is retiring (My oncologist said he could do my breast exams from here on out.)
- April 4 — Pre-Op abdominal/Pelvic CT scan and labs.
- April 7 — Labs, Checkup with oncologist.
- April 14 — Pre-Op appointment with plastic surgeon.
- April 26 — DIEP Flap Breast Reconstruction Surgery.
- April 26–May 1 — In ICU 2 nights, Burn unit 3 nights.
- April 30 — Chest CT scan.
- May 5 — Post-Op with plastic surgeon, Breast CT scan, Breast fluid test. Then back to plastic surgeon's office—lymph leak!
- May 6 — Return to plastic surgeon to check breast.
- May 9 — Follow-up with plastic surgeon.
- May 12 — Follow-up with plastic surgeon.
- May 23 — Follow-up with plastic surgeon.
- May 24 — Labs, Checkup with oncologist.
- June 13 — Brain MRI.
- June 21 — Lymphedema prevention follow-up.
- June 27 — Checkup with plastic surgeon.

- August 15 — Appointment with plastic surgeon to plan revision surgery, Lymphedema prevention follow-up.
- August 30 — Labs, Checkup with oncologist, Switched to Femara.
- September 12 — Bone Density Scan.
- October 13 — Checkup with radiation oncologist.
- December 1 — Labs, Checkup with oncologist, Prescribed Zoloft and Ativan.
- December 6 — Ambulance ride to Emergency Room after fainting. Head and chest CT scans, blood work, heart monitoring, 2-D doppler echocardiogram, doctor visits, and many other tests all day. Admitted into the hospital.
- December 7 — Brain MRI and continued doctor visits and tests. They ruled out all the scary stuff: no brain tumor, stroke, heart problems, seizures, blood clots.
- December 12 — Pre-Op appointment with plastic surgeon.
- December 21 — Breast revision surgery #1—Liposuction Fat Transfer.

2017

- January 3 — Follow-up with oncologist (I told him I'm feeling much better and had stopped the antidepressant shortly after I started it).
- January 9 — Post-Op with plastic surgeon.
- February 13 — Lymphedema prevention Follow-up.
- March 20 — Checkup with PCP, Prescribed Mobic to deal with bone pain.
- March 27 — Post-Op appointment with plastic surgeon.
- April 11 — Checkup with radiation oncologist.
- May 2 — Labs, Checkup with oncologist.
- May 9 — Diagnostic Mammogram and Sonogram for questionable lumps "all okay."
- June 12 — Pre-Op appointment with plastic surgeon.
- June 28 — Breast revision surgery #2—Liposuction Fat Transfer.
- July 10 — Post-Op appointment with plastic surgeon.
- July 24 — Checkup with plastic surgeon.
- August 8 — Labs, Checkup with oncologist, Switched from Femara to Aromasin.
- September 14 — Checkup with PCP, Referral to dermatologist.
- September 25 — Checkup with plastic surgeon.
- October 19 — Checkup with radiation oncologist.
- November 1 — First appointment with dermatologist.

- November 7 — Labs, Checkup with oncologist, Stopped Aromasin, Back on Nolvadex.
- November 27 — Pre-Op appointment with plastic Surgeon.
- December 8 — Breast revision surgery #3—Liposuction Fat Transfer.
- December 18 — Post-Op appointment with plastic surgeon.

2018

- January 8 — Checkup with plastic surgeon.
- March 29 — Nipple and Areola Tattooing.
- March 30 — Labs, Checkup with oncologist.
- May 2 — Brain MRI.
- July 30 — Labs, Checkup with oncologist.
- August 6 — Checkup with plastic surgeon.
- October 11 — Checkup with radiation oncologist.
- October 15 — Abdominal and pelvic CT scan to check out pelvic nodule "nothing serious."
- November 14 — Checkup with dermatologist, Biopsy of skin on back.
- November 21 — First appointment with physiatrist for underarm and shoulder pain "impingement syndrome of shoulder, acquired torsion dystonia," Referral to Lymphedema Physical Therapy.
- December 13 — Excision of pigmented nodular basal cell carcinoma on upper back.

2019

- January 24 — Nipple and Areola Tattooing touch-up.
- January 31 — Labs, Checkup with oncologist.
- February 12 — First of 12 appointments with Lymphedema PT (following Lymphedema PT appointments: February 25; March 1, 5, 8, 13; April 15, 24; May 7, 29; June 19; August 27).
- February 13 — Bone Density Scan.
- February 18 — Checkup with plastic surgeon.
- March 6 — Checkup with dermatologist.
- April 17 — Follow-up with physiatrist.
- May 24 — Diagnostic Colonoscopy "Precancerous Serrated Polyp, return in 5 years."
- July 17 — Checkup with dermatologist.
- July 30 — Labs, Checkup with oncologist.

- November 11 — Appointment with PCP's NP about shortness of breath, EKG Chest X-ray.
- November 13 — Checkup with dermatologist.
- November 22 — Stress Echocardiography.
- November 27 — D-Dimer Blood Test.
- December 4 — Complete Pulmonary Function Test.

2020

- January 17 — Chest CT scan, Call from PCP "Innumerable nodules in your lungs. It looks like the cancer is back."
- January 21 — Labs, including tumor marker CA27.29 "2,233 U/mL" (normal=<38 U/mL), Appointment with oncologist "Yes, the cancer is back; we need to test to see if it's breast cancer or a new cancer."
- January 27 — Liver Biopsy, Power Port Placement.
- January 30 — Labs, Treatment education with oncologist NP, "This is metastatic breast cancer," Meeting with cancer financial counselor.
- January 31 — Abraxane #1.
- February 3 — Checkup with plastic surgeon.
- February 7 — Labs, Checkup with oncologist NP, Abraxane #2.
- February 11 — Abdomonal/Pelvic CT scan, Whole Body Bone Scan.
- February 14 — Labs, Abraxane #3, "Cancer has spread to the liver, lymph nodes, possibly peritoneal and female organs."
- February 26 — First appointment with cancer psychologist.
- February 28 — Labs including tumor marker CA27.29 "1,197 U/mL" (normal=<38 UmL), Checkup with oncologist, Abraxane #4.
- March 6 — Labs, Abraxane #5, Started taking 1000mcg of B12 and 100mg of B6 daily for neuropathy.
- March 13 — Labs, Abraxane #6.
- March 27 — Labs including tumor marker CA27.29 "490 U/mL" (normal=<38 U/mL), Checkup with oncologist NP, Abraxane #7, First chemo alone as per coronavirus pandemic precautions, All workers wearing masks.
- April 3 — Labs, Abraxane #8.
- April 10 — Labs, Abraxane #9.
- April 24 — Labs including tumor marker CA27.29 "233 U/mL" (normal=<38 U/mL), Checkup with oncologist, Abraxane #10.
- May 1 — Labs, Abraxane #11.

- May 6 — Appointment with cancer psychologist via Telehealth.
- May 8 — Labs, Supposed to be Abraxane #12, but absolute neutrophil count (ANC) too low, Masks worn by all patients now.
- May 20 — COVID Test "result: not detected" (required now before each chemo cycle).
- May 21 — Labs including tumor marker CA27.29 "139 U/mL" (normal=<38 U/mL), Chest/Abdominal/Pelvic CT.
- May 22 — Appointment with oncologist "All tumors have shrunk and decreased in amount," Oncologist recommending Abraxane for 1 year vs. 6 months since my body has responded so favorably to it, Abraxane #12.
- May 29 — Labs, Abraxane #13.
- June 5 — Labs, Abraxane #14.
- June 17 — COVID Test "result: not detected."
- June 19 — Labs including tumor marker CA27.29 "77.6 U/mL" (normal=<38 U/mL), Appointment with Oncologist NP, Abraxane #15.
- June 26 — Labs, Abraxane #16.
- July 2 — Labs, Abraxane #17.
- July 15 — Telehealth appointment with cancer psychologist, COVID Test "result: not detected."
- July 17 — Labs including tumor marker CA27.29 "62.9 U/mL" (normal=<38 U/mL), Appointment with oncologist, Abraxane #18.
- July 24 — Labs, Abraxane #19.
- July 30 — Brain MRI "no cancer in the brain."
- July 31 — Labs, Abraxane #20.
- August 11 — Chest/Abdominal/Pelvic CT, COVID Test "result: not detected".
- August 14 — Labs including tumor marker CA27.29 "50.4 U/mL" (normal=<38 U/mL), Appointment with oncologist, "everything continues to improve, there is a new area in my neck to watch for possible cancer spread," Abraxane #21.
- August 21 — Labs, Abraxane #22.
- August 25 — Lymphedema prevention follow-up.
- August 28 — Labs, Abraxane #23.
- August 31 — Full body checkup with dermatologist.
- September 2 — Telehealth appointment with cancer psychologist.
- September 8 — COVID Test "result: not detected."
- September 11 — Labs including tumor marker CA27.29 "40.1 U/mL" (normal=<38 U/mL), Appointment with oncologist NP, Abraxane #24.

APPENDIX B

Suggested Bible Verses to Memorize When Battling Cancer

The LORD is the one who goes ahead of you; He will be with you. He will not fail you or forsake you. Do not fear or be dismayed.
    Deuteronomy 31:8

Have I not commanded you? Be strong and courageous! Do not tremble or be dismayed, for the LORD your God is with you wherever you go.
    Joshua 1:9

But You, O LORD, are a shield about me,
My glory, and the One who lifts my head.
I was crying to the LORD with my voice,
And He answered me from His holy mountain. *Selah.*
I lay down and slept;
I awoke, for the Lord sustains me.
    Psalm 3:3–5

In peace I will both lie down and sleep,
For You alone, O LORD, make me to dwell in safety.
    Psalm 4:8

The LORD also will be a stronghold for the oppressed,
A stronghold in times of trouble;
And those who know Your name will put their trust in You,
For You, O Lord, have not forsaken those who seek You.
    Psalm 9:9–10

The LORD is my light and my salvation;
Whom shall I fear?
The Lord is the defense of my life;
Whom shall I dread?
When evildoers came upon me to devour my flesh,
My adversaries and my enemies, they stumbled and fell.
    Psalm 27:1

I would have despaired unless I had believed that I would see the goodness of the LORD in the land of the living.
Wait for the LORD;
Be strong and let your heart take courage;
Yes, wait for the LORD.
    Psalm 27:13–14

You have turned for me my mourning into dancing;
You have loosed my sackcloth and girded me with gladness,
That my soul may sing praise to You and not be silent.
O LORD my God, I will give thanks to You forever!
    Psalm 30:11–12

Be strong and let your heart take courage,
All you who hope in the LORD.
    Psalm 31:24

Our soul waits for the Lord;
He is our help and our shield.
For our heart rejoices in Him,
Because we trust in His holy name.
Let Your lovingkindness, O LORD, be upon us,
According as we have hoped in You.
    Psalm 33:20–22

I sought the LORD, and He answered me,
And delivered me from all my fears.
    Psalm 34:4

The LORD is near to the brokenhearted
And saves those who are crushed in spirit.
    Psalm 34:18

Why are you in despair, O my soul?
And why have you become disturbed within me?
Hope in God, for I shall again praise Him
For the help of His presence.
    Psalm 42:5

God is our refuge and strength, a very present help in trouble.
    Psalm 46:1

As for me, I shall call upon God,
And the LORD will save me.
Evening and morning and at noon, I will complain and murmur,
And He will hear my voice.
    Psalm 55:16–17

Cast your burden upon the Lord and He will sustain you;
He will never allow the righteous to be shaken.
    Psalm 55:22

When I am afraid, I will put my trust in You.
In God, whose word I praise,
In God I have put my trust;
I shall not be afraid.
    Psalm 56:3–4a

I will cry to God Most High
To God who accomplishes all things for me.
    Psalm 57:2

Hear my cry, O God;
Give heed to my prayer.
From the end of the earth I call to You when my heart is faint;
Lead me to the rock that is higher than I.
For You have been a refuge for me,
A tower of strength against the enemy.
Let me dwell in Your tent forever;
Let me take refuge in the shelter of Your wings. *Selah*
    Psalm 61:1–4

My soul, wait in silence for God only,
For my hope is from Him.
He only is my rock and my salvation,
My stronghold; I shall not be shaken.
On God my salvation and my glory rest;
The rock of my strength, my refuge is in God.
Trust in Him at all times, O people;
Pour out your heart before Him;
God is a refuge for us. *Selah.*
    Psalm 62:5–8

You who have shown me many troubles and distresses
Will revive me again,
And will bring me up again from the depths of the earth.
    Psalm 71:20

I will meditate on all Your work
And muse on Your deeds.
Your way, O God, is holy;
What god is great like our God?
You are the God who works wonders;
You have made known Your strength among the peoples.
    Psalm 77:12–14

He who dwells in the shelter of the Most High
Will abide in the shadow of the Almighty.
I will say to the LORD, "My refuge and my fortress,
My God, in whom I trust!"
For it is He who delivers you from the snare of the trapper
And from the deadly pestilence.
He will cover you with His pinions,
And under His wings you may seek refuge;
His faithfulness is a shield and bulwark.
 Psalm 91:1–4

When my anxious thoughts multiply within me,
Your consolations delight my soul.
 Psalm 94:19

Oh give thanks to the LORD, for He is good,
For His lovingkindness is everlasting.
 Psalm 107:1

Then they cried out to the LORD in their trouble;
He saved them out of their distresses.
He sent His word and healed them,
And delivered them from their destructions.
Let them give thanks to the Lord for His lovingkindness,
And for His wonders to the sons of men!
Let them also offer sacrifices of thanksgiving,
And tell of His works with joyful singing.
 Psalm 107:19–22

He will not fear evil tidings;
His heart is steadfast, trusting in the Lord.
 Psalm 112:7

This is the day which the LORD has made;
Let us rejoice and be glad in it.
 Psalm 118:24

If Your law had not been my delight,
Then I would have perished in my affliction.
I will never forget Your precepts, for by them You have revived me.
    Psalm 119:92–93

Your word is a lamp to my feet
And a light to my path.
    Psalm 119:105

My eyes anticipate the night watches,
That I may meditate on Your word.
    Psalm 119:148

Our help is in the name of the LORD,
Who made heaven and earth.
    Psalm 124:8

I wait for the LORD, my soul does wait,
And in His word do I hope.
    Psalm 130:5

You have enclosed me behind and before,
And laid Your hand upon me.
    Psalm 139:5

The LORD is righteous in all His ways
And kind in all His deeds.
The LORD is near to all who call upon Him,
To all who call upon Him in truth.
    Psalm 145:17–18

Trust in the LORD with all your heart
And do not lean on your own understanding.
In all your ways acknowledge Him,
And He will make your paths straight.
    Proverbs 3:5–6

The name of the LORD is a strong tower;
The righteous runs into it and is safe.
    Proverbs 18:10

Behold, God is my salvation,
I will trust and not be afraid;
For the LORD God is my strength and song,
And He has become my salvation.
    Isaiah 12:2

The steadfast of mind You will keep in perfect peace,
Because he trusts in You.
Trust in the LORD forever,
For in God the LORD, we have an everlasting Rock.
    Isaiah 26:3–4

'Do not fear, for I am with you;
Do not anxiously look about you, for I am your God.
I will strengthen you, surely I will help you,
Surely I will uphold you with My righteous right hand.'
    Isaiah 41:10

'For I know the plans that I have for you,' declares the Lord, 'plans for welfare and not for calamity to give you a future and a hope. Then you will call upon Me and come and pray to Me, and I will listen to you. You will seek Me and find Me when you search for Me with all your heart.
    Jeremiah 29:11–13

Behold, I am the Lord, the God of all flesh; is anything too difficult for Me?
    Jeremiah 32:27

The LORD's lovingkindnesses indeed never cease,
For His compassions never fail.
They are new every morning;
Great is Your faithfulness.
"The Lord is my portion," says my soul,
"Therefore I have hope in Him."
    Lamentations 3:22–24

The Lord God is my strength,
And He has made my feet like hinds' feet,
And makes me walk on my high places.
    Habakkuk 3:19

"Come to Me, all who are weary and heavy-laden, and I will give you rest. Take My yoke upon you and learn from Me, for I am gentle and humble in heart, and you will find rest for your souls. For My yoke is easy and My burden is light."
  Matthew 11:28-30

Jesus said to her, "I am the resurrection and the life; he who believes in Me will live even if he dies."
  John 11:25

"These things I have spoken to you, so that in Me you may have peace. In the world you have tribulation, but take courage; I have overcome the world."
  John 16:33

For the mind set on the flesh is death, but the mind set on the Spirit is life and peace.
  Romans 8:6

And we know that God causes all things to work together for good to those who love God, to those who are called according to His purpose.
  Romans 8:28

For I am convinced that neither death, nor life, nor angels, nor principalities, nor things present, nor things to come, nor powers, nor height, nor depth, nor any other created thing, will be able to separate us from the love of God, which is in Christ Jesus our Lord.
  Romans 8:38–39

Now may the God of hope fill you with all joy and peace in believing, so that you will abound in hope by the power of the Holy Spirit.
  Romans 15:13

Therefore I run in such a way, as not without aim; I box in such a way, as not beating the air; but I discipline my body and make it my slave, so that, after I have preached to others, I myself will not be disqualified.
  I Corinthians 9:26–27

But we have this treasure in earthen vessels, so that the surpassing greatness of the power will be of God and not from ourselves; we are afflicted in every way, but not crushed; perplexed, but not despairing; persecuted, but not forsaken; struck down, but not destroyed; always caring about in the body the dying of Jesus, so that the life of Jesus also may be manifested in our body.
    2 Corinthians 4:7–10

Therefore we do not lose heart, but though our outer man is decaying, yet our inner man is being renewed day by day. For momentary, light affliction is producing for us an eternal weight of glory far beyond all comparison, while we look not at the things which are seen, but at the things which are not seen; for the things which are seen are temporal, but the things which are not seen are eternal.
    2 Corinthians 4:16–18

Brethren, I do not regard myself as having laid hold of it yet; but one thing I do: forgetting what lies behind and reaching forward to what lies ahead, I press on toward the goal for the prize of the upward call of God in Christ Jesus.
    Philippians 3:13–14

Be anxious for nothing, but in everything by prayer and supplication with thanksgiving let your requests be made known to God. And the peace of God, which surpasses all comprehension, will guard your hearts and your minds in Christ Jesus.
    Philippians 4:6–7

Let the peace of Christ rule in your hearts, to which indeed you were called in one body; and be thankful.
    Colossians 3:15

Yet you do not know what your life will be like tomorrow. You are just a vapor that appears for a little while and then vanishes away.
    James 4:14

Casting all your anxiety on Him, because He cares for you.
    1 Peter 5:7

About the Author

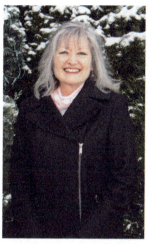

Camilla ("Camy") Adele (Stamps) Crank was born in Winfield, Kansas into a family wealthy in love. She graduated valedictorian from Arkansas City High School in 1978, received a Bachelor of Science degree in Health Care Administration with a Minor in Mathematics in 1982 from Wichita State University, graduating Magna Cum Laude—Go Shockers! Camy was employed by the Kansas Department of Social and Rehabilitation Services before marrying Captain Robert E. Crank and assuming her life-long occupation of wife and mother. Camy and Bob have been married for 37 years and have 3 adult children, 1 daughter-in-law, and 3 grandchildren. Camy says she fell in love with books while reading to her children, then became a writer when this book formed in her heart. You can contact her at camycrank@gmail.com. You can also follow Camy's cancer journey at https://www.caringbridge.org/visit/camycrank.

Made in the USA
Columbia, SC
14 May 2022